Comprehensive Atlas of High Resolution Endoscopy and Narrowband Imaging

EDITED BY

Jonathan Cohen MD, FASGE, FACG
Clinical Professor of Medicine
NYU School of Medicine
New York, NY, USA

FIRST EDITION

Blackwell
Publishing

© 2007 Blackwell Publishing Limited
Blackwell Publishing, Inc., 350 Main Street, Malden, Massachusetts 02148-5020,
USA
Blackwell Publishing Ltd, 9600 Garsington Road, Oxford OX4 2DQ, UK
Blackwell Publishing Asia Pty Ltd, 550 Swanston Street, Carlton, Victoria 3053,
Australia

First published 2007

2   2007

                    Library of Congress Cataloging-in-Publication Data
Comprehensive atlas of high resolution endoscopy and narrow band imaging / edited
by Jonathan Cohen. – 1st ed.
        p. ; cm. – (Advanced digestive endoscopy)
    Includes bibliographical references and index.
    ISBN-13: 978-1-4051-5886-2 (alk. paper) 1. Endoscopy–Atlases. I. Cohen,
Jonathan, 1964- II. Series.
    [DNLM: 1. Endoscopy, Gastrointestinal–methods–Atlases. 2. Gastrointestinal
Neoplasms–diagnosis–Atlases. WI 17 C736 2007]
    RC78. 7.E5C66 2007
    616.07′545–dc22   2007001193

ISBN: 978-1-4051-5886-2

A catalogue record for this title is available from the British Library
Set in 9/11.5pt Palatino by Charon Tec Ltd (A Macmillan Company), Chennai, India
Printed and bound in Navara, Spain by GraphyCems

Commissioning Editor: Alison Brown
Editorial Assistant: Jennifer Seward
Development Editor: Rob Blundell
Production Controller: Debbie Wyer
DVD produced by: Meg Barton and Nathan Harris

For further information on Blackwell Publishing, visit our website:
http://www.blackwellpublishing.com
The publisher's policy is to use permanent paper from mills that operate a sustainable
forestry policy, and which has been manufactured from pulp processed using acid-free
and elementary chlorine-free practices. Furthermore, the publisher ensures that the text
paper and cover board used have met acceptable environmental accreditation standards.

Contents

A companion DVD containing the text, images, and video clips is included at the end of the book.

Preface

Since the introduction of the flexible endoscope, physicians have been able to explore the images of the gastrointestinal (GI) tract in health and in disease, and use this information to make diagnoses and direct therapies. Over time, endoscopists have steadily been able to reach more locations and visualize the mucosa with increasing clarity.

Despite these advances, the advent of disruptive technologies is now raising uncertainty about the future of purely diagnostic endoscopy. In this context, the development of high-resolution endoscopy (HRE) and narrowband imaging (NBI) promises to breathe critically needed new value to the endoscopic examination of the GI tract. To survive as more than a solely therapeutic modality, endoscopy must evolve not only to provide better quality images than available by other new technologies, but also to reveal more useful diagnostic information than heretofore possible with standard optical imaging.

HRE and NBI stand out among new imaging modalities in a few ways. First, the incorporation of high-definition TV capability to endoscopy carries the prospect of general improvement in visualization throughout endoscopic practice. HRE alone may increase the detection rate of various pathologic findings, and the benefit of this advance to the average endoscopist should be immediate. NBI also has great promise in enhancing the specific diagnosis of certain conditions, and a number of studies that confirm this will be reviewed in the following chapters. What is most striking is how accessible this technology is likely to be for the general gastroenterologist to learn and incorporate into his or her practice.

While it will be relatively easy for endoscopists to purchase and start using HRE and NBI right away, it is clear that a comprehensive atlas of these images will be essential for them to fully understand what they are looking at and to maximize the benefit of this enhanced imaging capability.

This desire to provide a thorough guide to accelerate the learning curve for individuals wishing to adopt NBI HRE was the primary motivating force behind this volume. Emphasis is naturally placed on those conditions for which NBI is considered particularly useful, such as finding dysplasia in Barrett's mucosa and ulcerative colitis, and detecting adenomatous colon polyps. However, since HRE and NBI generate such dramatic new images throughout the GI tract, we aimed to provide a comprehensive look at the bowel using this lens. It is intended that the images selected for this volume will generate the excitement that resulted at each of the earlier major steps forward in endoscopic imaging technology. The reader will note that this atlas contains many images both from Japan and the UK using the LUCERA system and from throughout Europe and North America using the EXERA II system. Contributing centers will be noted for all photos, and differences between the two systems will be explained within the introductory chapters.

This book begins with a series of introductory chapters to review the theoretical framework for HRE and NBI, the historical development of this technology, the way it actually works, and the essential practical information needed to start using these endoscopes. The following section includes chapters looking at some of the proposed clinical applications of HRE and NBI along with preliminary supportive data, organized by organ system. Finally, the atlas contains color plates of images in high resolution white and narrowband light, in low and high magnification, along with correlating histopathology, to illustrate normal and abnormal pathology throughout the GI tract. For images shown without corresponding pathology photos, the pathology reports were reviewed by the contributing authors to ensure the accuracy of the descriptions within the captions. Particularly for those conditions in which NBI is felt to facilitate diagnosis, the atlas includes multiple examples, where possible, to illustrate the range of endoscopic findings. The accompanying DVD contains 55 video clips of diagnostic and therapeutic procedures to provide a more complete sense of how NBI works and looks in real time. This is fitting as this imaging modality is geared to enhance endoscopic decision-making in real time, to facilitate therapeutic maneuvers and to make tissue sampling more precise.

Admittedly, this field is in its early stages. The technology is still evolving and much investigation is ongoing to elucidate the usefulness of the findings. Many of the contributing authors to this volume are pioneers in developing this technology and in discovering the clinical implications of the patterns that are revealed. I am indebted to their efforts to collaborate on this project and help generate this atlas to rapidly disseminate their expertise and demonstrate the way endoscopy will look in the years to come.

Jonathan Cohen MD, FASGE, FACG
Clinical Professor of Medicine
NYU School of Medicine

Acknowledgments

The detailed explanations and images of NBI in the laryngopharynx (Dr. Muto), esophagus (Dr. Inoue), stomach (Dr. Yao and Dr. Kaise), and colon (Dr. Sano and Dr. Matsumoto) are abstracted from a book published in Japan, entitled "Atlas of New Endoscopic Imaging Technologies – Unique Diagnostic Imaging Using NBI, AFI and IRI", Nihon Medical Center, Inc. 2006 (edited by Hisao Tajiri). I am indebted to this publisher for the use of this material.

Special thanks are due to Dr. Brian West for his assistance in reviewing all pathology images and captions included in this volume. Additionally I would like to express my utmost thanks for the cooperation of Olympus America Inc. and Olympus Medical Systems Corp. In particular, I must single out the extraordinary effort of Eric Coolidge of Olympus in helping me coordinate many of the contributors worldwide to make this project possible. Finally, I wish to thank Paul Blaise and Stephen Holsapple of Blaise Media for their considerable help in editing the video material.

Companion DVD

The DVD accompanying this book contains:

- Video clips (these are referenced in the text)
- A searchable database of images from the book
- The complete text with a full text search.

Pathology Editor

A. Brian West MD, FRCPath
Director of Gastrointestinal Pathology
Services, AmeriPath New York
Gastrointestinal Diagnostics
Shelton, CT, and
Adjunct Professor of Pathology,
NYU School of Medicine, NY, USA

Contributors

Ajay Bansal
University of Kansas School of
Medicine, Kansas City,
MO, USA

Jacques Bergman
Academic Medical Center
University of Amsterdam
The Netherlands

Jonathan Cohen
NYU School of Medicine
New York, NY, USA

Guido Costamagna
Digestive Endoscopy Unit
Catholic University of the
Sacred Heart and
A. Gemelli University Hospital
Rome, Italy

Carmen Cuffari
The Johns Hopkins University
School of Medicine
Baltimore, MA, USA

Wouter Curvers
Academic Medical Center
University of Amsterdam
The Netherlands

Jacques Deviere
Erasmus University Hospital
Brussels, Belgium

James DiSario
University of Utah Health Sciences
Center, Salt Lake City,
UT, USA

James East
Wolfson Unit for Endoscopy
St. Mark's Hospital
UK

Paul Fockens
Academic Medical Center
University of Amsterdam
The Netherlands

Kazuhiro Gono
Research Department
Olympus Medical Systems Corp.,
Tokyo, Japan

Christopher Gostout
Mayo Clinic School of Medicine
Rochester, MN, USA

Gregory Haber
Lenox Hill Hospital
New York, NY, USA

Rob Hawes
Medical University of
South Carolina
Charleston, SC, USA

Fumihito Hirai
Department of Gastroenterology
Fukuoka University
Chikushi Hospital
Fukuoka, Japan

Mitsuo Iida
Department of Medicine and
Clinical Science
Graduate School of Medical Sciences
Kyushu University
Fukuoka, Japan

Haruhiro Inoue
Digestive Disease Center
Showa University Northern
Yokohama Hospital
Yokohama, Japan

Akinori Iwashita
Department of Pathology
Fukuoka University
Chikushi Hospital
Fukuoka, Japan

Makoto Kaga
Digestive Disease Center
Showa University Northern
Yokohama Hospital
Yokohama, Japan

Mitsuru Kaise
Department of Endoscopy
The Jikei University
School of Medicine
Tokyo, Japan

Philip Kaye
Department of Pathology
University Hospital
Queen's Medical Centre
Nottingham, UK

Shin-ei Kudo
Digestive Disease Center
Showa University Northern
Yokohama Hospital
Yokohama, Japan

Tetsuji Kudo
Department of Medicine and
Clinical Science
Graduate School of Medical Sciences
Kyushu University
Fukuoka, Japan

Guilherme Macedo
Servico de Gastrenterologia
Hospital Sao Marcos
Braga, Portugal

Toshiyuki Matsui
Department of Gastroenterology
Fukuoka University
Chikushi Hospital,
Fukuoka, Japan

Takayuki Matsumoto
Department of Medicine and
Clinical Science
Graduate School of Medical Sciences
Kyushu University
Fukuoka, Japan

Manabu Muto
Endoscopy & Gastrointestinal
Oncology Division
National Cancer Center
Hospital East
Chiba, Japan

Takashi Nagahama
Department of Gastroenterology
Fukuoka University
Chikushi Hospital
Fukuoka, Japan

Takashi Nakayoshi
Department of Endoscopy
The Jikei University
School of Medicine
Tokyo, Japan

Atsushi Ochiai
Pathology Division
National Cancer Center Research
Institute East
Chiba, Japan

Maria Oliva-Hemker
The Johns Hopkins University
School of Medicine
Baltimore, MD, USA

Ron Palmon
Mount Sinai School of Medicine
New York, NY, USA

Thierry Ponchon
Edouard Herriot Hospital
Lyon, France

Krish Ragunath
Wolfson Digestive Disease Centre
University Hospital
Queen's Medical Centre
Nottingham, UK

Douglas Rex
Indiana University School of
Medicine
Indianapolis, IN, USA

Jean-François Rey
Institute Arnault Tzanck
St Laurent du Var, France

Richard Rothstein
Dartmouth Hitchcock Medical Center
Lebanon, NH, USA

Yasushi Sano
Gastrointestinal Center
Sano Hospital
Kobe, Japan

Brian Saunders
Wolfson Unit for Endoscopy
St Mark's Hospital, UK

Yoshitaka Sato
Digestive Disease Center
Showa University Northern
Yokohama Hospital
Yokohama, Japan

Uwe Seitz
University Medical
Center Hamburg Eppendorf
Germany

Prateek Sharma
University of Kansas
School of Medicine
Kansas City, MO, USA

Nib Soehendra
University Medical Center
Hamburg Eppendorf
Hamburg, Germany

Suketo Sou
Department of Gastroenterology
Fukuoka University
Chikushi Hospital
Fukuoka, Japan

Satoshi Sugaya
Digestive Disease Center
Showa University Northern
Yokohama Hospital
Yokohama, Japan

Hisao Tajiri
Division of Gastroenterology
and Hepatology
Department of Internal Medicine
The Jikei University
School of Medicine
Tokyo, Japan

Hiroshi Tanabe
Department of Pathology
Fukuoka University
Chikushi Hospital
Fukuoka, Japan

Michael Wallace
Mayo Clinic School of Medicine
Jacksonville, FL, USA

Jerome Waye
Gastrointestinal Endoscopy Unit
Mount Sinai School of Medicine
New York, NY, USA

Herbert Wolfsen
Mayo Clinic School of Medicine
Jacksonville, FL, USA

Kenshi Yao
Department of Gastroenterology
Fukuoka University
Chikushi Hospital
Fukuoka, Japan

Shigeaki Yoshida
Director
National Cancer Center
Hospital East
Chiba, Japan

Part I

The Basics of NBI

Narrowband imaging: historical background and basis for its development

Shigeaki Yoshida

In Japan where the incidence of gastric cancer is very much higher than the rest of the world, greater attention has been paid to early diagnosis since the beginning of 1950s when the "gastrocamera" was first introduced. In those days, the finding of early gastric cancer (EGC) was not frequent and most of these lesions were identified from the differential diagnosis of deeply ulcerated (type III) or polypoid (type I) lesions, which can be easily detected. In 1970s, early diagnosis progressed and it became possible to detect those cancers showing the appearance of ulcer scar (type IIc) and plateau-like elevation (type IIa). In the beginning of 1980s, furthermore, early diagnosis of gastritis-like malignancy (IIb-like type) became more readily possible following the results of retrospective studies of rapidly growing advanced cancer [1]. With this increased appreciation of the appearance of early superficial lesions, widespread use of biopsy together with careful scrutiny of the mucosa using dye spraying techniques, EGCs which appear just as a faint mucosal irregularity or discoloration came to be the most frequent EGC that were being diagnosed by late in the 1980s [2].

Such results were applied also to esophageal and colorectal malignancies, and there has been a general acceptance in Japan that early malignancies in the alimentary tract may not appear polypoid or ulcerative. The desire to better recognize such malignancies, which may be difficult to distinguish from nonspecific inflammation or trauma, had prompted us to envision new endoscopic technology capable of revealing cancer-specific images in the surface structure of the mucosa. It is within this context that the field of narrowband imaging (NBI) was developed as a promising way to facilitate the endoscopic diagnosis of early neoplastic and pre-cancerous lesions in the alimentary tract.

NBI is an optical image enhancement technology that enhances vessels in the surface of mucosa and patterns of the surface of mucosa by employing the characteristics of light spectrum.

The development of NBI goes back to the study of spectroscopy in 10 years ago. The national project "Second Term Comprehensive 10-Year Strategy for Cancer Control" started in 1994. Together with Prof. N. Oyama of Tokyo Institute of Technology and Olympus Medical Systems Corp., we received funding from the project and started the study in which we intended to digitalize the color and structure of mucosa for the establishment of more objective/quantitative pathological diagnosis, hence for better diagnostic yield. At that time, multiple facilities and industries had conducted studies to realize optical biopsy using the characteristics of light spectrum. We aimed to achieve differentiation of normal and abnormal mucosa using a custom-made spectrophotometer developed by Olympus Medical Systems Corp.

By the method described in Figure 1.1, we obtained and analyzed more than 2,000 samples from esophagus, stomach and colon. However, we faced multiple challenges to establish a stable diagnostic standard. The spectrum showed different patterns in normal vs. abnormal tissues. But, the spectrum pattern differed from patient to patient, so that stable classification between normal and abnormal was quite difficult to summarize. Furthermore, spectrum data was not stable by the measuring conditions.

However, through the study, we noticed the specific pattern of spectrum when choosing certain narrow band wavelengths (Figure 1.2). To highlight the specific pattern, we shifted our study from qualitative data from spectroscopy to qualitative imaging that enhances details of the mucosal surface. As a result, when employing a narrow band filter, we found excellent light enhancement deep in the mucosa at red light wavelength, shallow mucosal surface at blue light wavelength and in between levels at green light wavelength [3]. Based on the findings, we continued study with the research and development group of Olympus and finally found that narrow band blue light wavelength matched the light absorption characteristics of blood hemoglobin and enhanced details of the mucosal surface.

In December 1999, we obtained the world's first clinical images using NBI in our facility (Figures 1.3–1.6). The original technology only generated black and white monochrome color with limited information for diagnosis, making it impractical for clinical applications. The challenge was shortly solved by the introduction of newer improved filters and the development of a prototype incorporating a circuit board exclusively for NBI color display.

Since these first clinical NBI pictures were achieved, we actively expanded the study in cooperation with multiple research facilities. As a result of this collaborative investigation, the application of NBI diagnosis expanded rapidly [4,5]. Starting with the diagnosis of colonic tumor and squamous cell carcinoma of esophagus, the applications of NBI were established in other fields such as superficial carcinoma in pharynx, Barrett's esophagus and adenocarcinoma, stomach cancer, and inflammatory bowel disease. Multiple studies were published in these areas; the results have been published in academic society proceedings, research committee reports and clinical papers in peer reviewed journals. Much of this data will be discussed in detail in subsequent chapters in this text.

In December 2005, the NBI system became commercially available from Olympus, and the technology and diagnosis expanded further, not only in Japan, but also worldwide.

In summary, endoscopic diagnosis has been rapidly progressing. Beyond technical advancement such as chromoendoscopy and improvement of image quality, endoscopic diagnosis is now advanced to the area of pathology. This is possible because the imaging technology now allows assessment of the three-dimensional architecture of tissue by fine examination of the mucosal surface with magnifying endoscopy. In the coming years, special light observation such as NBI may further be able to provide even more information about a targeted lesion, in order to clarify the indication of new cancer therapies.

Such endoscopic diagnosis through special light observation holds great promise. None of these advances could have been achieved without great contribution by Prof. H. Niwa, Board Chairman of the Japan Gastroenterological Endoscopic Society, and his colleagues who have devoted themselves to the development of multiple modalities of optical diagnosis, such as ultraviolet gastrocamera, infrared and auto-florescence imaging, since the project was first initiated while working together at Tokyo University in the past decade. We must recognize the history of endoscopic diagnosis and the contribution and diligences of these individuals in bringing the field to where it is today. I hope that special light diagnosis through NBI will become an increasingly reliable tool with more clinical evidence to support its applications. As this occurs, this technology should make important contributions to improve and facilitate diagnosis in clinical practice.

REFERENCES

1. Yoshida S, Yoshimori M, Hirashima T et al. Nonulcerative lesion detected by endoscopy as an early expression of gastric malignancy. *Jpn J Clin Oncol* 1981; 11: 495–506.
2. Yoshida S, Yamaguchi H, Tajiri H, et al. Diagnosis of early gastric cancer seen as less malignant endoscopically. *Jpn J Clin Oncol*. 1984; 14: 225–41.

3. Gono K, Obi T, Yamaguchi M et al. Appearance of enhanced tissue features in narrowband endoscopic imaging. *J Biomed Opt.* 2004; 9: 568–77.
4. Sano Y, Kobayashi M, Hamamoto Y, et al. New diagnostic method based on color imaging using narrowband imaging (NBI) endoscopy system for gastrointestinal tract. *Gastrointestinal Endoscopy* 2001; 53: AB125.
5. Kara MA, Fockens P, Peters F et al. Narrowband imaging (NBI) in Barrett's esophagus: what features are relevant for detection of high-grade dysplasia (HGD) and early cancer (EC)? *Gastroenterology* 2004; 126: A50.

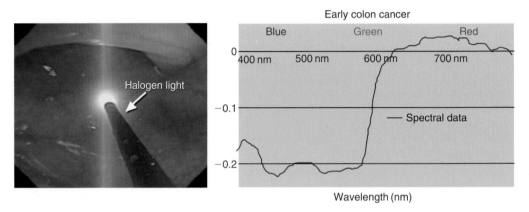

Figure 1.1 Spectral reflectance analysis. Spectral data were sampled at intervals of 2 nm ranging from 400 to 800 nm. In each examination, we measured spectral reflectance at both normal and neoplastic areas (Copyright S. Yoshida).

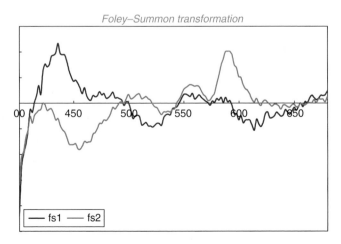

Figure 1.2 Spectral sensitivity functions for discrimination of cancerous regions (Copyright S. Yoshida).

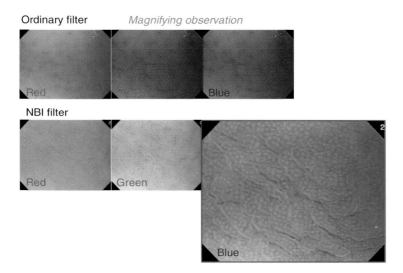

Figure 1.3 Normal gastric mucosa. Mucosal crypt pattern of the stomach could be observed without dye spraying by blue-filtering of NBI (Copyright S.Yoshida).

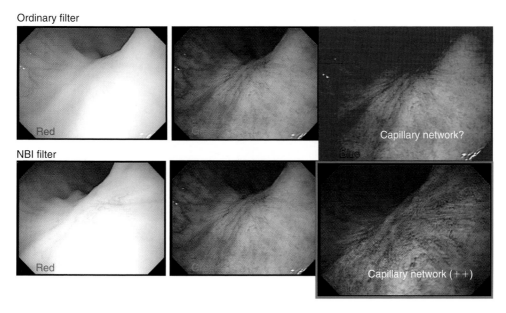

Figure 1.4 Gastric ulcer scar. Capillary network could be observed without dye spraying by blue-filtering of NBI (Copyright S.Yoshida).

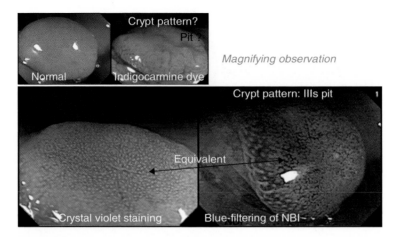

Figure 1.5 Flat adenoma of sigmoid colon. Crypt pattern of the depressed area could be observed without dye spraying by blue-filtering of NBI (Copyright S.Yoshida).

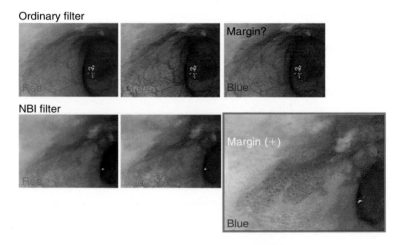

Figure 1.6 Esophageal cancer (type 0–IIc). The margin of lesion is clearly detected by blue-filtering of NBI (Copyright S.Yoshida).

An introduction to high-resolution endoscopy and narrowband imaging

Kazuhiro Gono

INTRODUCTION

The development of NBI (narrowband imaging) started in May 1999. To confirm the idea of NBI, a study using a multi-spectrum camera capable of producing spectroscopic images and high-power light source was conducted, with this author volunteering as a test subject. The study revealed that the use of 415 nm narrow band light can improve the contrast of capillary images which are difficult to observe under conventional white light. The first image of living tissue ever produced on NBI is shown in Figure 2.1. Then, the development of an NBI endoscopy system proceeded in cooperation with Dr. Sano of National Cancer Center Hospital East. On December 14, 1999, based on a study using the NBI prototype, we confirmed that the technology was promising for endoscopies of colon, stomach and esophagus.

Since this time, we have developed products in cooperation not only with Japanese, but also endoscopists from around the world in an effort to expand the capacity of the prototype. EXERA II, the next generation system equipped with both HDTV and NBI, was introduced in December 2005.

At present, Olympus has two types of video endoscopy systems in use worldwide. The difference between both systems is based on how a color image is produced. One is based on a color CCD chip which has several tiny color filters in each pixel. This system is the 100 series and is branded as EVIS EXERA II. The second system is based on a black and white CCD, in which color separation is achieved through the use of an RGB color filter wheel equipped within the light source unit. This system is the 200 series and is branded as EVIS LUCERA SPECTRUM. Both systems possess NBI technology. Research and development for NBI was first attempted with the EVIS LUCERA SPECTRUM system, the system predominant in Japan, UK, and Asian countries. Once success was achieved with that system, research and development was focused on the use of NBI with the color CCD system or EVIS

EXERA II. Both systems possess the same optical filter in the light source, which enables the illumination of two narrow-bands within the visible spectrum of light for NBI. As such, both systems are "optically" identical. However, since both technologies are fundamentally different, there are actually some minor differences in image reproduction. But for NBI, both systems are the same, as they both provide improved image contrast when viewing micro-vessel patterns within the superficial mucosa. If both systems images were compared simultaneously without magnification, some observers may notice slight differences. However, these differences are quite minor and have not been shown to be clinically significant.

Apart from these optical features, the two systems do differ in the method of magnification incorporated into the endo-scopes and the resulting capability to magnify the images observed. In the EXERA II system, the endoscope currently has digital zoom at 1.2 and 1.5 times magnification. The HDTV format also possesses "physical zoom" properties which allow the scope tip to be advanced up to 2 mm away from the mucosal surface without losing resolution. This combined feature results in a capacity for at least a 50-fold magnification. In contrast, the LUCERA system utilizes an optical zoom system, similar to that used in previous non-high-resolution zoom magnification endoscopes, that allows for magnification of the image up to 80 times. However, these numbers for mucosal magnification are somewhat limited in reliability, as there are a number of variables that may affect the actual magnification of tissue that is observed, such as the size of the monitor that is used.

HDTV is a video format that provides clear and high-resolution images while NBI offers high-contrast image of blood vessels. In theory, combining these technologies will give the best performance in the close observation of the mucosa. Knowing the design concept of the functions equipped with EXERA II, its technical limitations and how to read NBI images should be helpful in learning the practical use of HDTV and NBI.

There are many "High Definition" TV formats. At the time of product development, 1080i and 720p were the most popular as they still are today. Olympus had to consider which format would provide the highest level of resolution for motion and still imaging, as well as maintain its popularity within the market so current and future peripheral devices such as monitors, printers and digital recorders would remain compatible. As the result, 1080i was selected and has proven to be the most popular high definition broadcast format to this day.

Unlike conventional image processing, NBI is a technology in which an image is emphasized by light. Designing such light requires an in-depth understanding about optical characteristics of the living tissue. As an introduction, this chapter first discusses characteristics of light, including wavelength and color, as well as the interaction between the living tissue and light, such as absorption and scattering. Next, it describes the value offered by HDTV and NBI in terms of image quality and the method for designing chromatic image on NBI. Finally, this chapter will explain how typical endoscopic findings such as fine mucosal pattern and blood vessel images look on NBI and why they look that way, using illustrations.

LIGHT AND BIO-OPTICS

Light and wavelength

Light is an electromagnetic wave having both characteristics of wave and particle. When seeing light as a wave, the distance from peak to peak in each wave is called "wavelength" (Figure 2.2). Visible wavelength ranges from 400 to 700 nm. A different wavelength is perceived as a different color. Although colors look different depending on the psychological state of each individual, 400 nm, on average, is perceived as blue, 550 nm as green and 600 nm as red. Generally, saturation decreases when light contains more wavelengths. In other words, blue light having narrow bandwidth looks more vivid compared with that having broad bandwidth. Light having a broad bandwidth within the range between 400 and 700 nm looks white.

Color, absorption and reflection

When white light illuminates the surface of an apple, pigment in apple skin absorbs light ranging from 400 to 550 nm. The absorbed light is converted to heat. In other words, energy in the blue–green range from the white light is converted to heat. Unabsorbed light ranging from 550 to 700 nm is reflected. The reflected light reaches our eyes and the apple is perceived to be red. How would an apple look if cyanic colored light, instead of white, illuminates it? Cyanic colored light mainly consists of blue and green light, and because such light is absorbed by pigment and almost no light is reflected, the apple looks black. That is to say, white light is needed to perceive natural color of an object. Contrarily, the light does not need to be white if it is not intended to reproduce appearance of an object in natural color. NBI is based on this idea and developed for the purpose of highlighting blood vessels, not reproducing natural colors. Therefore, light other than white is used for NBI.

Light scattering

In relation to light propagation in an optical turbid medium such as diluted milk, light scattering needs to be taken into consideration in addition to reflection and transmission. Milk contains a number of fat globules of various sizes (1–100 μm). When light strikes such small particles, it diffuses three-dimensionally. This is called light scattering. When there are a multitude of particles, multiple scattering occurs as scattered light scatters again by striking another particle. Light propagates diffusively due to this light scattering even when a flux of light such as laser beam is injected into milk.

Absorption and scattering in tissue

A schematic diagram of the interaction between light and living tissue is shown in Figure 2.3. When light enters biological tissue, some reflects on the surface and some diffuses within the body. Multiple scattering occurs among light and small particles such as cell nuclei, cell organelles and nucleoli in the tissue. As a result, light propagates diffusively through the tissue. The propagation of light is determined by its wavelength. Red, having a long wavelength, diffuses widely and deeply, while blue, having a short wavelength, diffuses in a smaller range. This is shown in Figure 2.4.

A part of scattered light is absorbed by blood. To be accurate, hemoglobin absorbs blue and green light. Hemoglobin is a type of chromophore. Components in the gastrointestinal mucosa apart from hemoglobin, such as cell nuclei and fiber tissue, do not have colors. Therefore, the color of the gastrointestinal mucosa is mainly determined by hemoglobin.

The interaction between light and living tissue is characterized by hemoglobin, which strongly absorbs blue and green light and multiple scattering in biological tissue.

RESOLUTION AND CONTRAST

Resolution and contrast are terminologies to describe image quality. Figure 2.5 shows a relationship between resolution and contrast. A good quality image cannot be provided when resolution is high but poor in contrast. Image quality is the best when the level of both resolution and contrast is high.

Resolution is a term that describes a capacity to present minute patterns. Using the resolution chart in Figure 2.5 can define the capacity of an optical device, which is to reveal the fineness of detail in the chart. Resolution is determined by pixel numbers of CCD, signal processing and lens characteristics. Resolution of an endoscope capable of producing HDTV standard images is significantly greater than that attained using conventional endoscopes.

Contrast is defined as the ratio of density or brightness between a pattern and its background. The word describes clarity – how vividly the subject stands out against the background or the other way around. As shown in Figure 2.5, a pattern cannot be seen clearly when it is low in contrast, though superior in resolution. NBI is a technology capable of improving the contrast of blood vessels selectively. Resolution is enhanced by HDTV while NBI improves contrast. As a result, the combination of HDTV and NBI can offer a high-quality image of blood vessels analogous to the illustration in the above right of Figure 2.5.

BASIC PRINCIPLES AND SYSTEM DESIGN

Basic principles

Figure 2.6 is a schematic diagram of NBI. Two blood vessels running in living tissue are named BV(A) and BV(B), respectively. Broad band light composed of wavelengths of $\lambda1$, $\lambda2$ and $\lambda3$ is injected into BV(A) and narrow band light consists of wavelength $\lambda2$ is injected into BV(B). The degree of absorption into blood is $\lambda2 >> \lambda1, \lambda3$. $\lambda1$ and $\lambda3$ diffuse more widely and deeply within the tissue compared with $\lambda2$. When $\lambda2$ strikes the blood vessel, most of its energy is absorbed by blood. On the other hand, when $\lambda1$ and $\lambda3$ light rays strike the blood vessel, some of the energy transmits to the blood vessel and scatters deeply and widely. As a result, some of the scattered light rays of $\lambda1$ and $\lambda3$ re-transmit to the blood vessel or go around the blood vessel and exit from the mucosal surface. When the vessel is observed with an illumination containing light that is rarely absorbed by blood and scatters widely and deeply like $\lambda1$ and $\lambda3$, a blurry image as shown in VI(A) is produced. This is the conventional light source of endoscopes. On the other hand, when $\lambda2$ strikes the peripheral mucosa, the light is observed at the mucosal surface as scattered light without going around the blood vessel. As a result, the contrast of the blood vessel is improved as the vessel is indicated in black due to its strong absorbing capacity and in brighter colors for other parts as shown in VI(B). Figure 2.7(a) is an image of the blood vessel pattern of the underside of the human tongue mucosa illuminated by conventional broad band blue light. Figure 2.7(b) is an image produced by narrow band blue light. By changing the illumination to narrowband, we can see that the contrast of the capillary patterns of Figure 2.7(a) is improved in Figure 2.7(b). NBI is a technology to observe biological tissue with narrow band light, created by extracting wavelengths that are strongly absorbed by blood and do not diffuse widely and deeply from the conventional broad band light.

System design

Figure 2.8 shows blood vessel images of the underside of the human tongue mucosa produced by narrow band light of 415, 500, 540 and 600 nm. A very fine pattern of the blood vessel is reproduced by the 415 nm light and a thicker pattern is indicated by the light with a longer wavelength. Blood vessels in the tongue mucosa are believed to become finer at the superficial layer of the mucosa as shown in lower figure of Figure 2.8. The relationship between blood vessel images and these narrow band illuminations is provided in the figure. It is most appropriate, by the principle of NBI, to choose 415 nm to observe capillaries on the surface and 540 nm for thicker vessels. On the other hand, blood vessels in the deeper part are reproduced in the 600 nm image. However, considering the fact that early cancer develops on the superficial layer and changes the blood vessel structure there, using 600 nm images in NBI can only make a small contribution to medical applications. Therefore, NBI system uses two narrow band illuminations of 415 and 540 nm.

Figure 2.9 shows the configuration of the NBI system in the EVIS EXERA II system. A xenon lamp is installed in front of an optical filter for NBI. It is a double-band filter (415 and 540 nm) as described previously. When observing with NBI, the filter is placed on the light path. Under normal observation, the filter is removed from the optical axis. Under NBI observation, the light from the xenon lamp splits into two bands (415 and 540 nm) and the split light illuminates the mucosa.

As shown in Figure 2.9, two narrow band images of 415 and 540 nm are reproduced when the NBI filter is placed. However, in order to create color images, we need three images to be outputted to R, G and B channels of the monitor. There are variations as to which bandwidth goes to which channel, but in order to achieve high visibility of blood vessels, first, the capillary patterns on the superficial layer of the mucosa need to be reproduced as a black and white pattern, and second, the relatively thick vessels in the deeper part of the mucosa need to be highlighted with a color different from that of the capillary pattern. Therefore, colors are allocated according to human visual perception.

Man finds it easier to perceive a very fine pattern with luminance (Figure 2.10 Pattern A) rather than colors (Figure 2.10 Pattern B). Thicker vessels can be perceived easily with a color pattern (Figure 2.10 Pattern C). Considering such characteristics, 415 nm is allocated to B and G channels so that the blood vessels on the surface are reproduced in a brownish pattern much like black and white pattern, and 540 nm is allocated to R channel so that the vessels in the deeper part are indicated in a cyanic color pattern (Figure 2.11).

Blood vessels and bleeding

When observing the mucosal surface closely with an HDTV scope, capillaries on the superficial layer of the mucosa are seen as brownish pattern on NBI (Figure 2.12(a) lower figure). When a blood vessel is thin and CCD is unable to produce its image clearly, it is reproduced as a blurry, brownish spot. Relatively thick blood vessels located in the deeper part of the mucosa are reproduced in cyanic hue.

On the other hand, bleeding is shown in black, tar-like color, because light rays of 415 and 540 nm are absorbed by blood on the mucosal surface and not reflected.

In many tumors, blood vessel density on the superficial layer of the mucosa becomes high. In case of esophageal squamous cell carcinoma, for example, expansion, growth and meandering of intrapapillary capillary loops (IPCLs) are findings characteristic of the disease. These are visibly perceived as brownish areas when observed by NBI from middle-long distance (Figure 2.12(a) upper figure).

Fine mucosal pattern

Figure 2.12(b) shows a cross-sectional diagram of the colonic mucosa. Micro-vessels running in the tissue between the crypt foci are reproduced in brownish hue since they are the same as capillaries on the mucosal surface shown in Figure 2.12(a). On the other hand, no materials around the crypt foci absorb light except cells surrounding the gland. Therefore, a significant amount of light is reflected and the crypt foci are presented in a white pattern. As a result, the fine mucosal pattern of the large bowel is reproduced as a brown–white pattern. Gastric mucosa and Barrett's mucosa, both having a similar gland structure, are also presented in the same way. NBI is expected to produce an effect similar to chromoendoscopy. NBI can highlight the fine mucosal pattern as long as mucus is transparent, which does not exert influence over observation. On the other hand, when capillaries are not developed in the tissue between the crypt foci as seen in hyperplastic polyps, the fine mucosal pattern is not highlighted on NBI.

Squamo-columnar junction

Stratified squamous epithelium of the normal esophageal mucosa has few blood vessels and reflects light strongly when seen optically. Therefore, it is presented as a bluish white image on NBI. On the other hand, for the surface of the gastric mucosa, having a number of blood vessels, the whole mucosa is observed in brownish hue. Therefore, the esophageal mucosa and gastric mucosa at the SCJ are reproduced in a strong contrast of white and brown (Figure 2.12(c)). The extent of Barrett's mucosa, like normal squamo-columnar junction (SCJ), can be detected easily with the contrast of the normal esophageal mucosa. Detecting the normal esophageal epithelium surrounded by Barrett's mucosa would especially be easier compared with the normal observation.

Residue and bile

Residue and bile in the large bowel are reproduced in yellow hue under white light. The yellow pattern is presented in red (as if bleeding) on NBI. Residue and bile strongly absorb the 415 nm light while reflecting the 540 nm light strongly. Since NBI produces 540 nm images on R channel and 415 nm images on B and G channels of the output monitor, images on B and G channels become darker while those on R get brighter on the monitor. Therefore, residue and bile are indicated in the color of blood red.

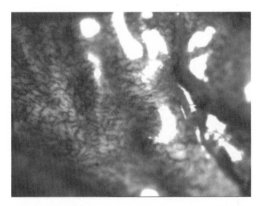

Figure 2.1 The 415 nm narrow band image of human tongue mucosa. The 415 nm narrow band image reflects fine capillary pattern on the mucosa which has been hard to be visualized under conventional white light (Copyright K. Gono).

Wavelength

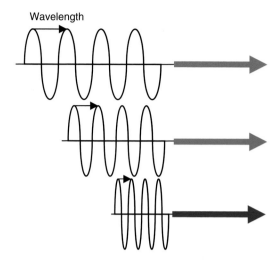

Figure 2.2 Wavelength and related color. Wavelength is defined as the distance from peak to peak in each wave. Longer wavelength has the appearance of reddish and shorter one shows bluish appearance (Copyright K. Gono).

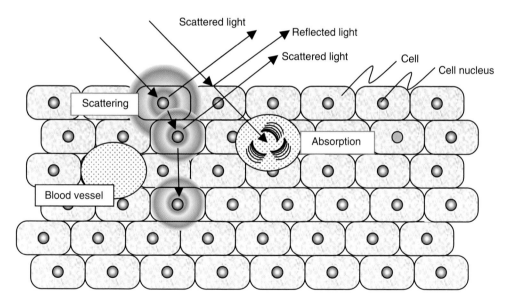

Figure 2.3 Interaction between light and biological tissue (Copyright K. Gono).

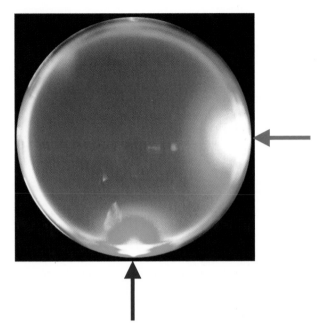

Figure 2.4 Diffusively light propagation in turbid medium. Red light diffuses in the turbid medium widely and deeply, while blue light does not diffusively propagate (Copyright K. Gono).

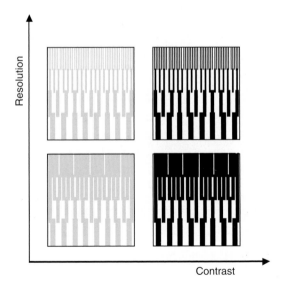

Figure 2.5 Contrast vs. resolution. Resolution in here means the resolution of CCD used for imaging resolution chart (Copyright K. Gono).

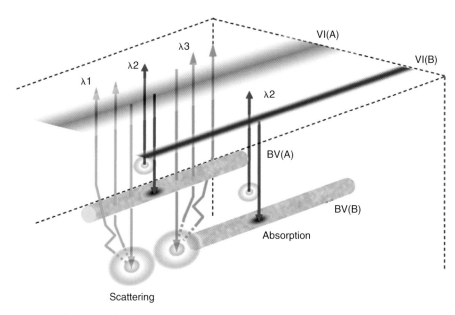

Figure 2.6 Contrast of blood vessel (Copyright K. Gono).

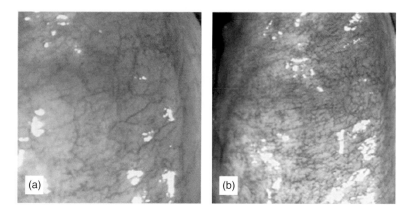

Figure 2.7 Blood vessels of human tongue. (a) Image under conventional broad band blue light. (B) Image under narrow band blue light (Copyright K. Gono).

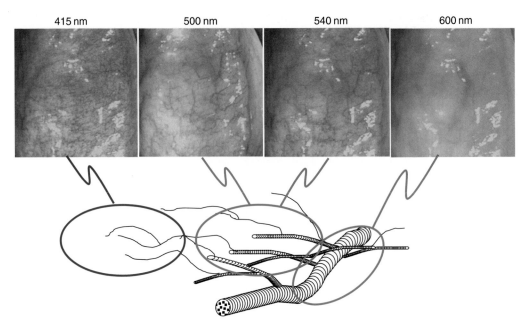

Figure 2.8 Endoscopic images of human hypoglottis mucous membrane (Copyright K. Gono).

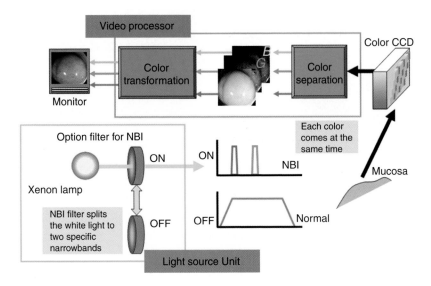

Figure 2.9 Structure of NBI system (Copyright K. Gono).

Pattern A   Pattern B   Pattern C

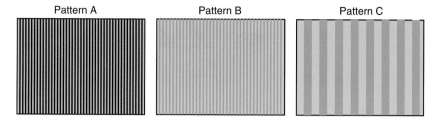

Figure 2.10 Human visual perception to black and white pattern and color pattern (Copyright K. Gono).

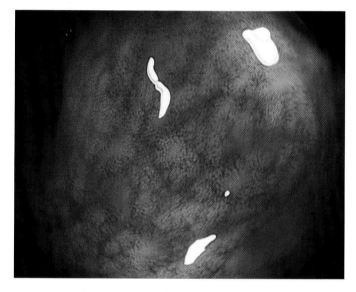

Figure 2.11 Appearances of endoscopic findings on NBI endoscopy. Fine superficial capillaries appear brown whereas the deeper vessels appear cyanic in color. Image courtesy of Jonathan Cohen (NYU Medical Center).

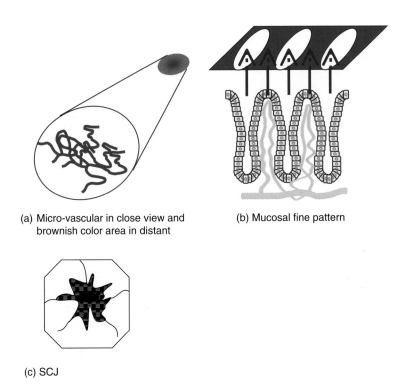

(a) Micro-vascular in close view and
brownish color area in distant

(b) Mucosal fine pattern

(c) SCJ

Figure 2.12 Application of NBI (Copyright K. Gono).

Getting started with high-resolution endoscopy and narrowband imaging

3

Ajay Bansal and Prateek Sharma

INTRODUCTION

The advent of newer imaging modalities such as high-resolution endoscopy (HRE) and narrowband imaging (NBI) represents an immense improvement over the current standard white light endoscopy. HRE is a technologically advanced method of endoscopic imaging that provides a high-quality image by using a much higher number of pixels (1 million) than the conventional endoscopes. NBI uses narrow spectra of blue light (440–460 nm) and green light (540–560 nm). This results in good visualization of superficial details of the mucosa. The detailed mechanisms of these two technologies are discussed elsewhere. However exciting the new technology, there will be a significant but not insurmountable learning curve associated with familiarizing oneself with the working visualization and interpretation of findings provided by the new imaging techniques. The following few sections will introduce the endoscopist to the basic use of HRE/NBI technology, but the only way to improve recognition of patterns is initial training and then regular performance of HRE/NBI endoscopy.

THE HRE/NBI ENDOSCOPES

The HRE/NBI endoscopes are similar to the currently used endoscopes with the same tactile feel except for novel functions of various buttons on the endoscope. These cannot be used with a standard processor and require a special processor to be fully functional. HRE endoscopes function similar to the conventional endoscopes differing only in the quality of the image. The NBI endoscopes have a few specific features the user needs to be acquainted with (Figure 3.1). This chapter will refer primarily to the 180 series EVIS EXCERA II system utilized in the US and Europe. By the switch of a button, it can convert white light images to NBI images and vice versa. Depress another switch and the image can be digitally magnified. Each press of the switch changes the magnification with a maximum magnification of 1.5×. The magnification function in endoscopes is identical to the optical and digital zoom functions of commercially available cameras where the quality of a magnified image will be maintained by the optical zoom where a new set of lenses come into play while the digital zoom will artificially magnify the already captured image. On the 240 and 260 series LUCERA endoscopes utilized in Japan, optical magnification is achieved via a continuous elevator-like dial on the endoscope head. The LUCERA prototype NBI system does therefore have an optical zoom capability but the 180 series endoscopes provide only digital zoom. This digital magnification may not be always useful as the resolution of the image does not improve commensurate with the magnification. It remains to be seen whether or not such digital magnification makes a clinically relevant difference to the visualization of the mucosal and vascular details.

PREPARING THE PATIENT

During regular white light endoscopy, macroscopic abnormalities are examined whereas during NBI, the mucosal pattern and subtle changes are sought. Observing these finer minute details of the mucosa and the blood vessels with HRE and NBI requires a great deal of patient cooperation, much more so than with standard white light endoscopy. This requires a well-trained and experienced nurse who can keep the patient adequately sedated through the entire duration of the procedure. This may seem like a minor issue but occasionally, agitation on part of the patient makes it harder to maintain the NBI image in focus and prolongs the procedure. Effective communication with the sedation staff is a key to ensure adequate sedation and cooperation of the patient.

THE CAP TECHNIQUE

Ideally NBI of the esophagus should be performed by affixing a cap to the distal tip of the endoscope (Figure 3.2). The cap is a distal attachment (Olympus, disposable distal attachment; # D-201-1180) that is transparent and maintains a distance of 2–3mm between the mucosa and the tip of the endoscope. This helps obtain a well-focused image. Secondly, it helps keep the area of the mucosa in the field of vision for the details to be evaluated by the endoscopist. The cap will give the tip of the endoscope a wider dimension that may sometimes make the esophageal intubation tricky, but with practice and patience, the endoscope with the fitted cap can be advanced into the esophagus with fair ease. The procedure can be performed without a cap but the mucosal and vascular details may be difficult to appreciate, especially when starting.

PREPARING THE ESOPHAGUS

A major challenge in performing and evaluating the esophagus is that of mucus/oral secretions within the esophagus that may interfere with obtaining clear images. This can be tackled by adequate washes with water to clear the surface of the mucosa. If water rinses do not get rid of the mucus, then 10–20 ml of 50% N-acetylcysteine can be sprayed with the help of the spray catheter to clear the mucus. It is critical that the esophagus is as clean as possible before detailed inspection is carried out.

Peristalsis of the esophagus can make the performance of HRE/NBI difficult as the image can get in and out of focus. The cap technique may help with this. Also, use of an anti-peristaltic agent may diminish esophageal motility but has to be balanced against the potential side effects of the drug. At present, we do not use any anti-peristaltic agent in our practice. One such agent is butylscopolamine that has been approved for use in Europe and has been extensively used with confocal endoscopy that requires a still esophagus[1]. Butylscopolamine has a similar mechanism of action as scopolamine but a much shorter half-life (20 minutes vs. 2–3 hours with scopolamine). The potential side effects are primarily anticholinergic such as glaucoma exacerbation, urinary retention, blurry vision, dry mouth and confusion, but such significant side effects related to the drug have not been reported. With time and experience, esophageal motility may prove to be a minor issue with NBI. Nevertheless, the effect of this drug on visualization during NBI has never been studied.

EXAMINING THE ESOPHAGUS

Initially, a high-resolution white light examination should be performed to identify any visible lesions such as nodules, ulcers and plaques. All of these lesions will be highlighted during NBI but their visualization under white light may help perform a more focused NBI examination. Another reason to do a thorough examination under white light is to ensure that no obvious lesions are missed since we are all familiar with white light and using NBI will definitely have a learning curve to appreciate things under blue light. During this part of the procedure with white light, the mucosal surface should be thoroughly washed using multiple rinses of water to expedite the subsequent NBI portion that is more technically challenging.

An important issue is that all biopsies should be deferred to the end of the procedure, as presence of blood will interfere with the NBI examination.

Once the white light examination of the esophagus, stomach and duodenum is performed in the standardized manner, the user switches to NBI. This is accomplished by pushing a button on the top of the handle of the endoscope. The initial NBI examination should be performed with the optical magnification of 1× to ensure that there is no loss of resolution of mucosal architecture. The duodenal mucosa (Figure 3.3), antrum, body and fundus can then be examined followed by gradual withdrawl from the stomach till the circular pattern of the cardia (Figure 3.4) at the gastroesophageal junction is visualized. While focusing on this cardiac pattern and taking a cue by the proximal margin of the gastric folds, the endoscopist will notice a distinct change in the mucosal pattern that should coincide very closely to the end of the gastric folds. In a patient with Barrett's Esophagus (BE), this change in the mucosal pattern would be a transition into a ridge/villous pattern, suggestive of intestinal metaplasia. The identification of the proximal margin of the gastric folds is the traditional way of identifying the distal aspect of BE segment. But, in fact, although not formally reported, the change in the mucosal pattern from circular to ridge/villous may be better at identifying the extent of BE segment distally.

The first step is to examine the entire BE segment looking for macroscopic lesions not visualized on HRE and making a note of the abnormality by describing the level in centimetre and the quadrant of the esophagus. This will help revisit the lesions for subsequent biopsies. Under white light, blood appears red but during NBI, it looks pitch black and hence, a biopsy prior to a complete NBI examination will affect the assessment of the patterns adversely due to the introduction of blood. After the initial overview examination of BE is completed, then is the time to pay attention to the mucosal and vascular details that are seen due to the contrast provided by NBI, as well as the magnification function of the endoscope. Mentally, the examiner should try to focus on the two aspects of the examination – mucosal surface and vascular pattern. Finding an abnormal mucosal pattern should prompt search for abnormal vascular patterns and vice versa and it is possible that in the same area, either one of the pattern is clearer and distinct from the other. Every abnormal area should be noted in terms of location and biopsied separately to permit later correlation and mapping of the extent of dysplasia. After the NBI examination is complete, targeted as well as random biopsies can be obtained [see DVD video clip 11].

EXAMINING THE STOMACH, DUODENUM AND COLON

Like the esophagus, the duodenum and colon present relatively narrow lumen environments in which there is sufficient light to perform a complete visual survey of the mucosa under NBI light. This kind of examination mainly takes advantage of the contrast afforeed by the NBI image to facilitate detection of abnormalities that might appear subtle on white light examination. In the duodenum and colon, the novice quickly learns to recognize the appearance of bilious fluid and residual stool as pink in color. Limitations of a poor colon prep create the same difficulties for a NBI examination as with a standard colonoscopy.

Unlike these narrow lumen organs, the stomach has a relatively wide lumen, and there often is not enough light to perform a proper initial scan for abnormalities under NBI light but could be used for close up study of areas of interest.

As with the esophagus, after the initial scan to detect possible abnormalities, any suspicious lesion elsewhere in the gastrointestinal tract can be viewed by NBI to examine the mucosal pattern and the microvessels in an attempt to characterize the lesion and determine its extent. In this regard, motility can be an issue, as with the esophagus.

VARIOUS PATTERNS OBSERVED BY NBI

The following few paragraphs will discuss the patterns of NBI in BE patients as an example of how specifically NBI is applied in the gastrointestinal tract. The reader is referred to individual chapters for detailed NBI patterns of the esophagus, stomach and colon, and preliminary data supporting the utility of this imaging modality in detecting lesions and making endoscopic diagnoses in these organs.

Normal patterns

What are the "normal" patterns visualized in a BE segment without dysplasia? The intestinal metaplasia within the BE segment appears as a regular ridge/villous pattern (Figure 3.5). This appears as alternate longitudinal bands of dark and light areas. Some areas of the BE segment appear to have a circular pattern and these areas have a higher likelihood of harboring cardiac-type mucosa [2]. The normal vascular pattern on NBI in BE is comprised of regularly branching, uniformly organized small vessels. This should be differentiated from the larger caliber palisading vessels in the distal esophagus that are usually well visualized under white light examination.

Abnormal patterns

Knowing the normal patterns will help the endoscopist diagnose abnormal lesions. The most worrisome pathology in flat
BE mucosa is high-grade dysplasia/esophageal adenocarcinoma (HGD/EAC). This is manifested by irregular mucosal
patterns characterized by patterns of varying shapes, lengths
distributed unevenly giving a non-uniform look to the mucosa
(Figure 3.6). This is obviously a subjective description and is
the primary reason for the initial training. The BE segment
may need to be examined multiple times before the beginner
achieves a reasonable degree of skill to detect the most clinically relevant lesions of HGD/early EAC. Numerous examples
of both non-dysplastic and dysplastic Barrett's appearance on
NBI can be found within Chapter 6 and in the Atlas section in
Chapter 11. [see DVD video clip 13].

The vascular pattern is comparatively harder to decipher
than the mucosal pattern presumably as the process of angiogenesis may result in various sizes and shapes of vessel formation. Nevertheless, abnormal vascularity appears as increased
number, tortuous, dilated, corkscrew-type small blood vessels
of varying caliber. Others have described abnormal vascularity
in multiple ways with two descriptions that particularly cor-
relate well with presence of HGD – spiral vessels of varying
caliber and small isolated blood vessels [3]. For the future, a
uniform classification system of mucosal and vascular patterns
needs to be devised.

REFERENCES

1. Kiesslich R, Gossner L, Goetz M, Dahlmann A, Vieth M, Stolte M, Hoffman A, Jung M, Nafe B, Galle PR, Neurath MF. In vivo histol-ogy of Barrett's esophagus and associated neoplasia by confocal laser endomicroscopy. *Clin Gastroenterol Hepatol* 2006; 4: 979–987.
2. Sharma P, Bansal A, Mathur S, Wani S, Cherian R, McGregor D, Higbee A, Hall S, Weston A. The utility of a novel narrow band imaging endoscopy system in patients with Barrett's esophagus. *Gastrointest Endosc* 2006; 64: 167–175.
3. Kara MA, Ennahachi M, Fockens P, ten Kate FJ, Bergman JJ. Detection and classification of the mucosal and vascular patterns (mucosal morphology) in Barrett's esophagus by using narrow band imaging. *Gastrointest Endosc* 2006; 64: 155–166.

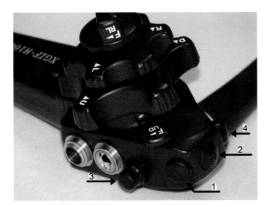

Figure 3.1 Function of the various switches on the NBI endoscopes: (1) switch to NBI from white light, (2) digital magnification (1× to 1.5×) and (3 and 4) to freeze and capture the image.

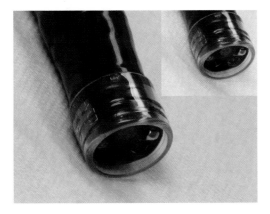

Figure 3.2 NBI endoscope with disposable distal attachment (inset shows a close up view).

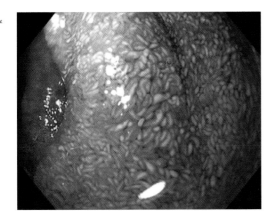

Figure 3.3 Duodenal villi (white) in the background of red (bile).

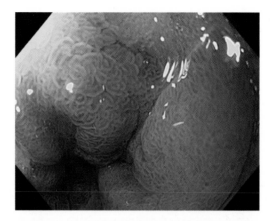

Figure 3.4 Circular pattern of the cardiac-type mucosa.

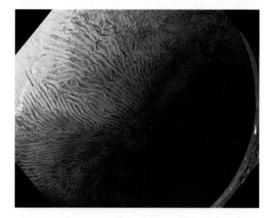

Figure 3.5 Ridge/villous pattern comprised of alternating longi-tudinal darker and lighter areas. This is suggestive of intestinal metaplasia.

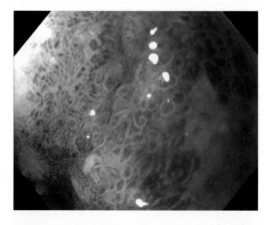

Figure 3.6 Irregular/distorted pattern of high-grade dysplasia.

Part II

Potential Applications of NBI and Early Supportive Data

Section 1

Pharynx and Esophagus

Detection of superficial cancer in the oropharyngeal and hypopharyngeal mucosal sites and the value of NBI at qualitative diagnosis

4

Manabu Muto, Atsushi Ochiai and Shigeaki Yoshida

WHY IS A DIAGNOSIS OF PHARYNX NECESSARY?

The clinical care of the pharynx is generally carried out by otolaryngologists. For this reason, many gastrointestinal (GI) physicians do not fully inspect and make diagnoses in the area of the oropharynx and hypopharynx during routine endoscopy. At the same time, it has been recognized difficult to detect an early cancer in the oropharyngeal and hypopharyngeal mucosal sites, because most cancer in this region is found in an advanced stage with several symptoms such as dysphagia and severe pains. The organ of the pharynx is essential to life and daily life by transferring food and liquid, and by breathing and phonation. Once the cancer is found in progress, patients lose these functions and patients' quality of life becomes indeed remarkably poor. Needless to say, detection of cancer in early stage is very much appreciated.

NBI (narrow band imaging) is a new technology developed in the field of GI endoscopy. Since we reported the value of NBI in combination with magnifying endoscopy for the detection of cancer in oropharyngeal and hypopharyngeal mucosal sites at first, importance in the diagnosis of the oropharyngeal and hypopharyngeal mucosal sites are more and more recognized [1]. In other words, a momentum for the detection of cancer in oropharyngeal and hypopharyngeal mucosal sites in early stage has been gained during upper GI endoscopy. And, the diagnosis of cancer in early stage is expected to contribute to patients' quality of life and improve their prognosis by enabling minimally invasive therapy to spare the organs, and thereby preserve function.

CHAPTER 4

CANCER IN THE AREA OF PHARYNX AND ITS RISK FACTOR

According to the report in 2003 by the Japan Foundation for Promotion of Cancer Research, new cancer cases in Japan exceed 500,000 in all areas [2]. The number of new cancer cases in the area of oral cavity and pharynx is 8,687 (1.7% of total cases) that is, approximately 1/12 of the cases of gastric cancer (101,379; 20.1% of total cases). Most of the cancers generated in oropharyngeal and hypopharyngeal mucosal sites are squamous cell carcinoma. Alcohol drinking and smoking have been recognized as two major risk factors as well as in the esophagus. In a recent study, it is implied that accumulation of acetaldehyde, the first metabolite of ethanol, is closely linked to carcinogenesis. Especially, in Asian people including Japanese, there is genetic polymorphism in aldehyde dehydrogenase type 2 (ALDH2), an enzyme responsible for the elimination of acetaldehyde. Heterozygotes for inactive gene (ALDH2-2) will have a higher risk of carcinogenesis when they keep drinking [3]. In other words, the one with a tendency of blushing at drinking (flushing response) is at higher risk for esophageal and pharyngeal cancer.

SUPERFICIAL CANCER IN OROPHARYNGEAL AND HYPOPHARYNGEAL MUCOSAL SITES

Current guidelines for head and neck cancer do not include an exact definition of superficial cancer [4]. In Japan where there is a high incidence of squamous cell carcinoma, the guideline for esophageal cancer considers a cancer up to submucosa as "superficial cancer" and a cancer invading beneath muscularis propria as "advanced cancer" [5]. Among superficial cancers, one up to epithelium or lamina propria mucosae without lymph node involvement or metastasis is defined as "cancer in early stage". There is no definition of invasion in the field of pharyngeal cancer except for carcinoma in situ (Tis) that reflects pathological invasion. According to statistics by Japan's Head and Neck Cancer Society in 2001 with 29 hospitals, carcinoma in situ counted only 1 case among 218 cases of hypopharyngeal cancer and no cases among all cases of oropharyngeal cancer [6]. Accordingly, it is recognized as extremely difficult to detect carcinoma in situ in oropharyngeal and hypopharyngeal mucosal sites. Generally, carcinoma in situ is recognized as a tumor with no risk of lymph node metastasis. When prognosis is taken into consideration, a definition linked to lymph node metastasis should be necessary. Histological diagnosis in this area should be studied further. Therefore in this chapter, high-grade intraepithelial neoplasia as defined in World Health

Organization (WHO) classification is regarded as "carcinoma in situ" and a cancer slightly invaded beneath epithelium as "superficial cancer"(Figures 4.1–4.4).

DIAGNOSIS OF SUPERFICIAL CANCER IN OROPHARYNGEAL AND HYPOPHARYNGEAL MUCOSAL SITE BY NBI

It is now safe to say that the era of GI endoscopy has changed from realistic diagnosis with white light and dye to the diagnosis of biological change using special light observation. Especially for neoplastic lesions, in the past, diagnosis had relied on the buildup between lesions and the surrounding area, and the change in color representing reddening and orange tone. Now using the properties of special light, the rationale of diagnosis has been changing, supported by the observation of biological change. NBI employs selectively filtered bandpass at 415nm that is well absorbed by hemoglobin. Therefore, NBI provides endoscopic images with fine capillary patterns and detailed observation of changes in the mucosal surface, especially when combined with high-resolution imaging and magnification (Figures 4.5–4.9).

We have studied NBI images of superficial head and neck cancer in aspects of "visibility" and "character of image" in combination with magnified endoscopy [7,8]. In terms of visibility, NBI displays cancerous areas as having a brownish appearance, so that a border between the lesion and normal mucosa can be clearly identified. In contrast, it is difficult to identify the border by normal white light observation. NBI clearly displays abnormal angiogenesis in a speckled form that is distinctively found in the lesion. In histology, this abnormal angiogenesis is similar to the morphological changes of intra-papillary capillary loop (IPCL) within squamous epithelium used to improve diagnosis in the esophagus, as will be described in detail in Chapter 5 of this volume [9].

1 Change in color defining areas at NBI observation (brownish area)
Superficial cancer tends to be displayed as brownish area at NBI observation. Superficial cancer with reddening can be identified under normal white light observation. However, NBI can display the border between a lesion and normal mucosa with or without reddening. The surface of normal squamous epithelium is seen as whitish with luster. In contrast, NBI displays lesions with tumorous change as a brownish area and shows a clear border between the lesion and the normal surrounding mucosa.

Benign lesions such as inflammation and basal cell hyperplasia often appears as a slight extension and generation of subtle vessels, but its interspersion do not comprise a well demarcated area. For example, a lesion with an abnormal change in IPCL but more diffuse interspersion is less likely to be cancerous. Conversely, a lesion that is seen as occupying a wide area but with a blurry IPCL change and a ground glass appearance also tends to have a benign etiology such as inflammation.

2 Change in IPCL shape

The size of the IPCL in normal epithelium is about $10 \mu m$. But, its size turns to $100 \mu m$ in cases of cancerous lesions. IPCL changes by extension, prolongation and meandering. Extension and prolongation reaches to the surface of epithelium so that they are clearly observed endoscopically. The number of vessels also increases within the lesion and beneath the epithelium. However, there are multiple patterns of changes in IPCL shape even within a lesion. Within carcinoma in situ, there are multiple patterns in angiogenesis among lesions. There are studies about the IPCL patterns in the esophageal field for the relationship to cancer invasion and histological staging which will be discussed in Chapter 5. But, the field of oropharynx and hypopharynx would tend to be different from the esophagus because the muscularis mucosae does not exist in the pharyngeal area. Further study is needed regarding the implications of IPCL patterns in the pharynx [see DVD video clips 1–8].

REFERENCES

1. Muto M, Nakane M, Katada C, et al. Squamous cell carcinoma in situ in oropharyngeal and hypopharyngeal mucosal sites. *Cancer* 2004; 101: 1375–1381.
2. Foundation for Promotion of Cancer Research: Statistics of Cancer '03. pp. 46–47, 2004 (only available in Japanese).
3. Yokoyama A, Kato H, Yokoyama T, et al. Genetic polymorphisms of alcohol and aldehyde dehydrogenases and glutathione S-transferase M1 and drinking, smoking, and diet in Japanese men with esophageal squamous cell carcinoma. *Carcinogenesis* 2002; 23: 1851–1859.
4. Japan Society of Head and Neck Cancer. *Clinical Guideline for Head and Neck Cancer* (3rd version). Kanehara Shuppan, Tokyo, 2001 (only available in Japanese).
5. Japan Esophageal Society. *Clinical Guideline for Esophageal Cancer* (9th version). Kanehara Shuppan, Tokyo, 1999 (only available in Japanese).
6. Japan Society for Head and Neck Cancer Registry Committee. Report of Head and Neck Cancer Registry of Japan, clinical statistics and registered patients, 2001. *Japan J Head Neck Cancer* 2005; 31: 60–80.
7. Muto M, Ugumori T, Sao Y, et al. Narrow band imaging combined with magnified endoscopy for the cancer at the head and neck region. *Dig Endosc* 2005; 17: S23–S24.

8. Muto M, Katada C, Sano Y, et al. Narrowband imaging: a new diagnostic approach to visualize angiogenesis in the superficial neoplasm. *Clin Gastroenterol Hepatol* 2005; 3: S16–S20.
9. Inoue H, Honda T, Nagai K, et al. Ultra-high magnification endoscopic observation of carcinoma in situ of the oesophagus. *Dig
Endosc* 1997; 9: 16–18.

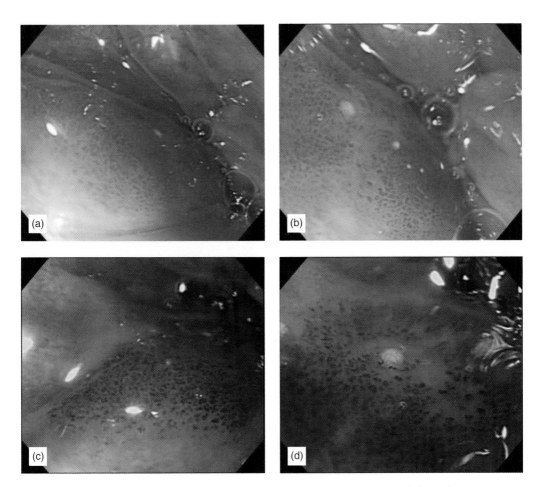

Figure 4.1 Carcinoma in situ in left piriform sinus. (a, b) Lesion exists in left piriform sinus
with intensive reddening (white light observation). (c, d) Compared to normal white light observation, the lesion is displayed clearly as a brownish area by NBI. Intensive speckle-like angiogenesis is clearly seen by NBI combined with zoom endoscopy. Intensive angiogenesis is clearly seen
by NBI combined with zoom endoscopy.

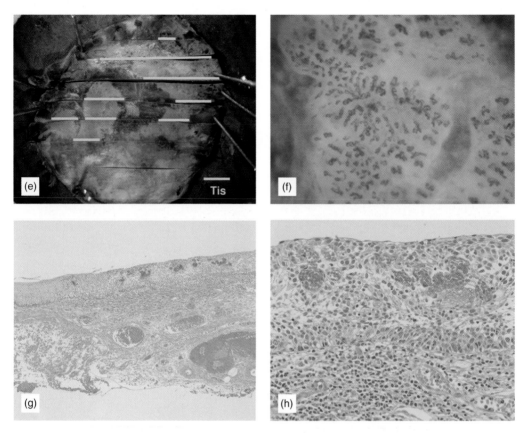

Figure 4.1 (Continued) (e) Iodide-dyed specimen obtained by endoscopic resection
under general anesthesia. Carcinoma in situ is identified in area not stained by iodide. (f)
Stereomicroscopic view of angiogenesis in area not stained by iodide. Angiogenesis unevenly
extends and the mucosal lesion not stained by iodide represents "pinky color". Angiogenesis
appears pink and clearly extends unevenly and displays a meandering, serpiginous shape. (g, h)
H&E view of specimen obtained by EMR. (g) Low magnification of squamous cell carcinoma in
situ. (h) High magnification extended IPCL is identified within carcinoma in situ (Copyright M.
Muto, A. Ochiai, S. Yoshida).

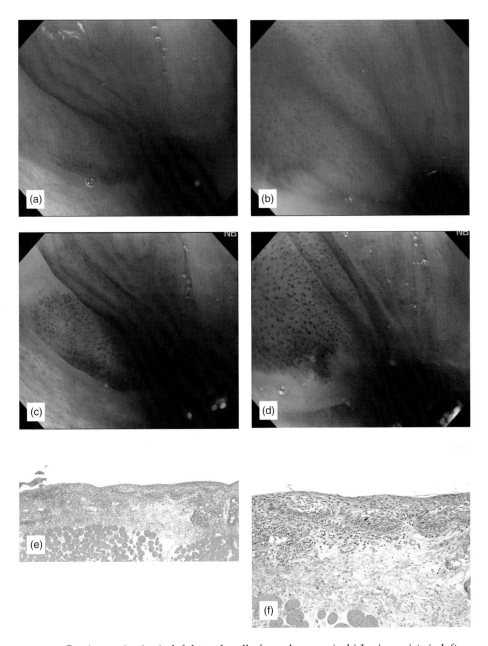

Figure 4.2 Carcinoma in situ in left lateral wall of oropharynx. (a, b) Lesion exists in left lateral wall of the oropharynx. Area with slight reddening can be identified but, it is hard to identify its dimension. Partially, melanotic change is observed. It is a general tendency to see this in the area around superficial cancer in head and neck. Slight dot-type reddening identified by zoom endoscopy. (c, d) Compared to white light observation, this lesion can be clearly identified using NBI as a brownish area. Especially, the border in melanosis is clearly seen. NBI frequently displays melanotic change as brownish area. In such cases, careful observation is needed. Zoom endoscopy clearly shows extension and prolongation of angiogenesis. (e, f) H&E view of specimen obtained by EMR. (e) Low magnification. Squamous carcinoma in situ. (f) High magnification – Partially, melanin pigment is identified (Copyright M. Muto, A. Ochiai, S. Yoshida).

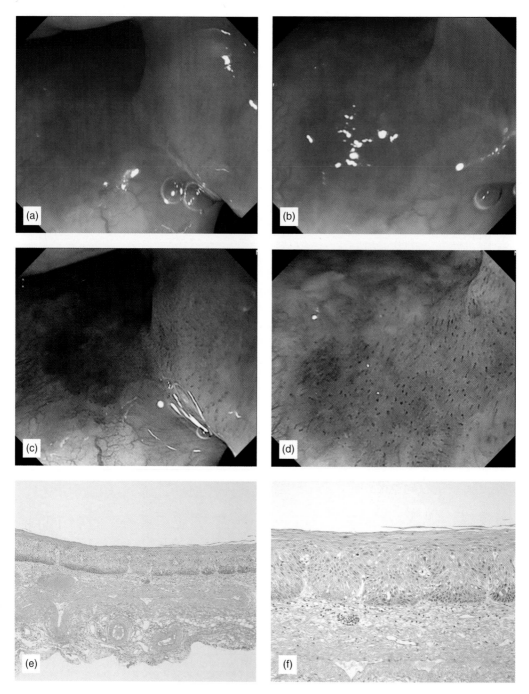

Figure 4.3 Carcinoma in situ at right side of vallecula epiglottica. (a, b) Lesion exists at right side of vallecula epiglottica. Vanishing vessels, slight reddening in the area and whitish mucosa at right base of tongue are identified. Reddening with luster in the area of vessel vanishes at zoom endoscopic view. (c, d) Area displayed in brownish by NBI matches with area vessel vanished in the right side of the vallecula epiglottica. At the right base of the tongue, a short slight whitish elevation is identified. Dot-like angiogenesis in a brownish area is identified under zoom endoscopy. (e, f) H&E view of specimen obtained by EMR. (e) Low magnification squamous carcinoma in situ within epithelium. (f) High magnification (Copyright M. Muto, A. Ochiai, S. Yoshida).

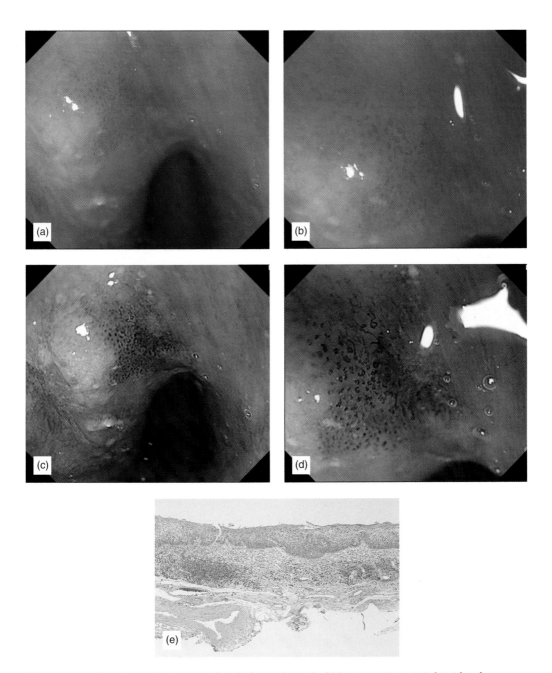

Figure 4.4 Carcinoma in situ at right piriform sinus. (a, b) Lesion exists at right side of piriform sinus. Slight reddening is identified. Angiogenesis and vessel extension in reddening area is identified under zoom endoscopy. (c, d) Lesion is clearly identified as a brownish area by NBI. Uneven prolongation and extension in brownish are identified under zoom endoscopy. (e) H&E view of specimen obtained by EMR. Squamous carcinoma in situ. The lesion is 5 mm in diameter and stays within the epithelium (Copyright M. Muto, A. Ochiai, S. Yoshida).

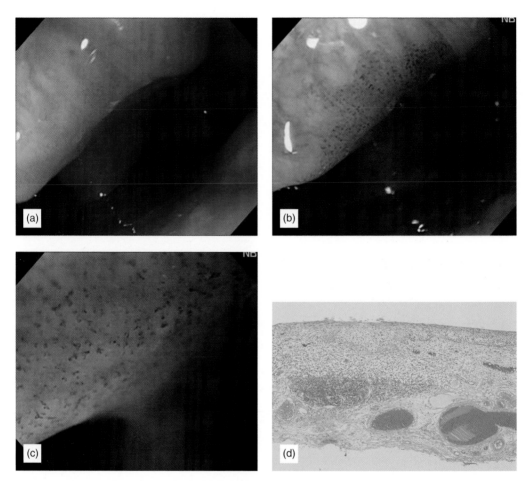

Figure 4.5 Superficial cancer at right piriform recess. Comparison between normal white light and NBI observation. (a) Lesion exists in right piriform recess. But, it is difficult to identify with normal white light observation. (b) Brownish area clearly separated by border is seen by NBI observation. (c) Uneven angiogenesis identified in brownish area under zoom endoscopy. (d) H&E view of specimen obtained by EMR. Squamous carcinoma in situ slightly invading beneath epithelium. Depth of tumor is 200 μm from the surface (Copyright M. Muto, A. Ochiai, S. Yoshida).

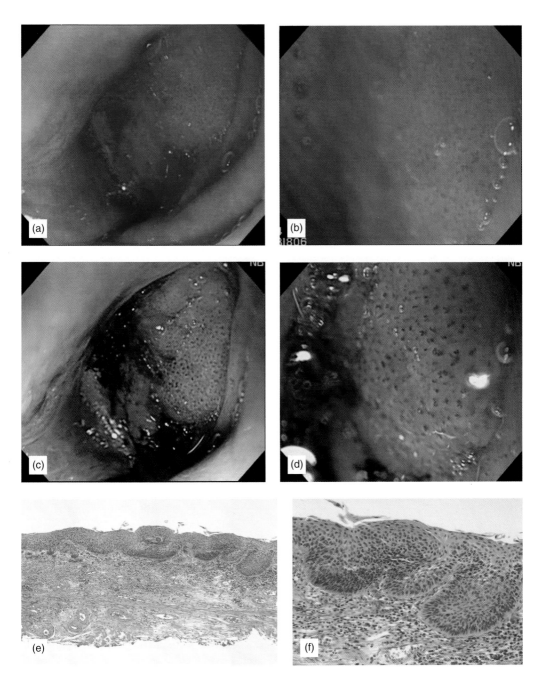

Figure 4.6 Carcinoma in situ at right piriform sinus. (a) Lesion exists at right piriform sinus. Short flat protrusion and easy friability. (b) Angiogenesis is identified under zoom endoscopy. (c) Identification of brownish area is difficult by NBI, but intensive dot-like pattern is identified. (d) Uneven angiogenesis with prolongation and extension like frog eggs are identified under zoom endoscopy. (e, f) H&E view of specimen obtained by EMR. (e) Squamous carcinoma in situ within epithelium. (f) High cell density. Angiogenesis is not remarkable (Copyright M. Muto, A. Ochiai, S. Yoshida).

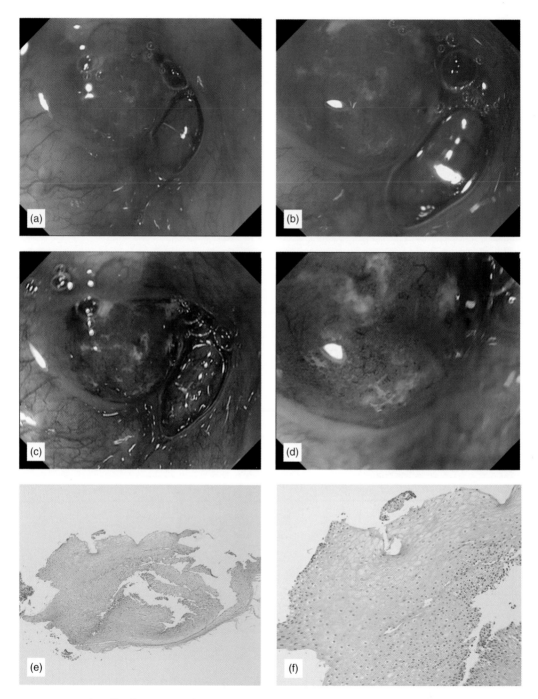

Figure 4.7 Small inflammatory lesion at vallecula epiglottica. (a) Slight reddening with vanishing vessel identified by normal white light observation. (b) Only reddening and erosion are identified under zoom endoscopy. (c) Color change to brown is identified by NBI. (d) Angiogenesis is not identified under zoom endoscopy. (e, f) H&E view of specimen. Concluded to be squamous epithelium with inflammatory infiltration (Copyright M. Muto, A. Ochiai, S. Yoshida).

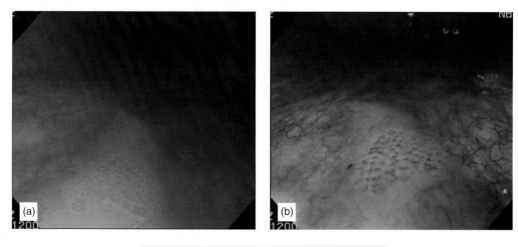

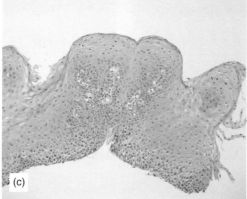

Figure 4.8 Small lesion at posterior wall of oropharynx. (a) Dimple-like lesion with rough surface somehow identified. (b) Dimple-like lesion with rough surface is identified by NBI. Difference from surrounding normal mucosa is not remarkable. Only shows slight thickness. (c) H&E view of specimen. Concluded to be squamous epithelium with low-grade papilla-like growth (Copyright M. Muto, A. Ochiai, S. Yoshida).

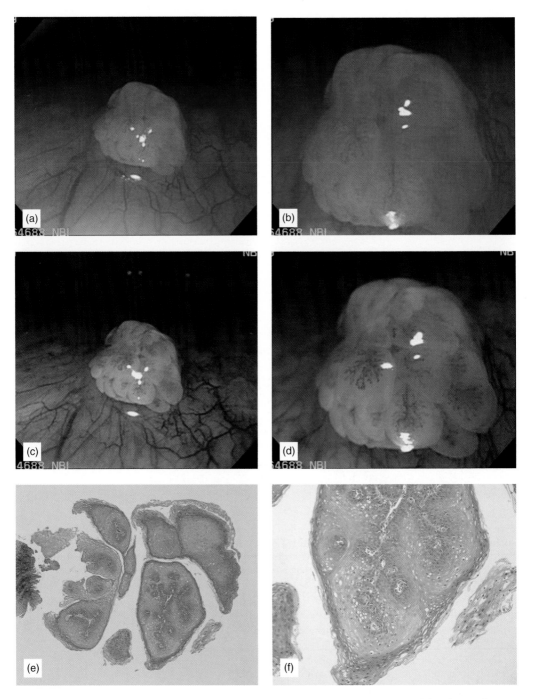

Figure 4.9 Papilloma at posterior wall of oropharynx. (a) Whitish pine-cone-like elevated lesion is identified. (b) Surface pattern and slight prolongation is identified under zoom endoscopy. (c) Papillary pattern is clearly identified from distance. Angiogenesis with prolongation inside papilloma slightly identified. (d) Fern-leaf-like prolonged angiogenesis is identified within papillary pattern under zoom endoscopy. (e, f) H&E view of specimen. Papillary propagation in squamous epithelium. Concluded to be a papilloma (Copyright M. Muto, A. Ochiai, S. Yoshida).

Magnifying endoscopic diagnosis of tissue atypia and cancer invasion depth in the area of pharyngo-esophageal squamous epithelium by NBI enhanced magnification image: IPCL pattern classification

5

Haruhiro Inoue, Makoto Kaga, Yoshitaka Sato, Satoshi Sugaya and Shin-ei Kudo

BACKGROUND

As methods to improve the prognosis of pharyngeal and esophageal cancer patients, we are conducting the following two strategies. One is detecting them in early stage and treating them by EMR/ESD (endoscopic mucosal resection/ endoscopic submucosal dissection) [1,2]. In other words, our goal is to detect early stage carcinoma during the endoscopic screening [3]. If you have an ability to detect a 1 mm neoplasia, then you would hardly overlook the 5 or 10 mm neoplasia. The other strategy is to conduct minimally invasive treatments according to the stage in which the lesion was detected. Once the lesion is detected, accurate diagnosis for the stage is performed, and the minimally invasive treatment which is not detrimental to the therapeutic effort is selected. The current standard medical guideline for the esophageal cancer is summarized in the "esophageal cancer treatment guideline in Japan". It states that for cases of mucosal carcinoma without lymph node metastasis, EMR should be applied. According to the strategy of *"en bloc* resection", we apply EMR to the lesion which is less than 2 cm and ESD using a triangular-tip knife to the lesion which is more than 2 cm in diameter. As to the lesion in which cancer invasion is deeper than sm2 (200 μm or more), we would select surgical esophageal resection and reconstruction due to the significant increased risk of lymph node involvement in such cases [4]. We would like to improve the prognosis for the esophageal cancer patient through early stage detection and to keep the quality of life high level by selecting the appropriate less invasive treatment according to disease staging.

It has been widely accepted that performing a standard endoscopic examination is mandatory for estimating the invasion depth of a lesion roughly which is either mucosal cancer or sm invasive cancer before the treatment. Furthermore, magnifying endoscopic observation is an additional tool that can support depth diagnosis with regular endoscopic diagnosis. On the other hand, the strongest argument for magnifying endoscopy is the diagnosis of irregular micro-vascular patterns within flat lesions (more likely an early stage lesion).

Stratified squamous epithelium in the pharynx and esophagus has no pit pattern which is routinely observed in glandular epithelium in stomach and colon. Magnifying endoscopy allows an observation of micro-vascular structure in the squamous epithelium. In the squamous epithelium, intra-epithelial papillary capillary loop (IPCL) is observed by magnifying endoscopy [5]. IPCL demonstrates characteristic changes in its figure according to the tissue atypism and cancer invasion depth [6]. IPCL type classification is directly related to the tissue characterization of a minute lesion [7].

When the lesion is diagnosed by biopsy specimen as a low-grade intraepithelial neoplasia (category III in Vienna classification [8]), careful follow-up has been recommended. In contrast, high-grade intraepithelial neoplasia (category IV in Vienna classification) endoscopic resection by EMR/ESD is recommended. For tiny lesions, endoscopic bite biopsy is difficult to perform.

MAGNIFICATION OF NORMAL ESOPHAGEAL MUCOSA

We describe the superficial capillary pattern of the normal esophageal mucosa and submucosa in Figure 5.1. When you approach normal mucosa without magnification, branching vessel network is observed which appears most commonly in the plane immediately above the muscularis mucosae. The IPCL (Figure 5.2), which rises perpendicularly from the branching vessel, is barely recognizable under normal observation of normal epithelium. By using the magnifying scope such as GIF-Q160Z and GIF-Q240Z, which has magnification capability up to 80 times, the normal mucosa of the IPCL is identified as red dots.

Narrowband imaging (NBI) enables more vivid observation of the IPCL. Branching vessels which are located at the relatively deeper layer are observed as green, and IPCL, which is located at more superficial layer, is observed as brown loops (brown dots) (Figure 5.5).

DIAGNOSTIC PROCESS OF MUCOSAL CANCER

Screening for mucosal cancer

Early cancer detection is directly related to less invasive treatment. If a lesion is found as mucosal cancer instead of submucosal cancer, it can be treated by EMR/ESD rather than surgery because mucosal cancer usually has no risk of lymph node metastasis. Therefore, the purpose of screening endoscopy is to find mucosal cancer.

We have been reporting that the changing pattern of the IPCL through magnifying endoscopic observation in the squamous esophagus is extremely useful for tissue characterization and diagnosis of carcinoma invasion depth. In the esophageal squamous epithelium, we consider that the change in the IPCL pattern reflects the structure irregularity (shape change of epithelial papilla) caused by carcinoma. NBI enhances blood vessels sharply.

MAGNIFYING ENDOSCOPIC DIAGNOSIS OF IPCL PATTERN IRREGULARITY IN THE ESOPHAGEAL SQUAMOUS EPITHELIUM

In carcinoma of the esophageal squamous epithelium, four characteristic changes in IPCL pattern are found in the non-iodine-stained part. Those are dilation, meandering, caliber change and uneven form in each IPCL (Figure 5.3). Changes in the IPCL progress start from healthy mucosa, inflammation, dysplasia and finally to cancer.

Actual diagnosis consists of two steps. The first step is to detect the lesion as a brownish area or as non-iodine-stained lesion. The next step is to observe the suspected area with high magnification and then evaluate the IPCL pattern (Figure 5.4).

It is categorized from Type I (normal mucosa) to Type V (carcinoma). Type II is often equivalent to regenerative tissue or inflammation, Type III is a border line lesion which is often related to low-grade intraepithelial neoplasia, Types IV and V are equivalent to high-grade intraepithelial neoplasia, and Type V-1 is reflecting carcinoma (Figures 5.5–5.9). We consider that this reflects the structural irregularity of the tissue. In Type IV, changes in IPCL are simple in structure, when compared to the significant changes in Type V-1. However, under newly developed NBI processing, IPCL change is more easy to observe and differentiate because NBI creates a noticeable contrast of vascular system from background tissue.

It is significant that the endoscopic diagnosis of flat mucosal lesions is possible by classifying the IPCL pattern in the magnified image. We have been judging that endoscopically the IPCL Type III needs to be surveyed periodically, while tissue with higher than IPCL Type IV needs to be treated through EMR/ESD.

INVASION-DEPTH DIAGNOSIS STANDARDS FOR SUPERFICIAL CARCINOMA (BASED ON THE CHANGE IN IPCL)

In standard endoscopy without magnification, depth diagnosis is estimated mainly by observation of the concavity of the lesion and/or the degree of the uplift, change of color tone and change in the shape by air insufflation. Because diagnosis of sm massive invasive cancer is actually sufficient by normal observation alone, the depth diagnosis for the cancer by magnifying endoscopy is considered as supplemental information to these above-mentioned conventional criteria.

In the depth diagnosis by magnifying endoscopy, changes in the IPCL and the appearance of neoplasm blood vessels become the criteria for assessing depth. Although IPCL shows changes that include four characteristic factors at m1, as it advances to m2 and m3, destruction of IPCL advances gradually (Type VN) and these changes are further extended into the submucosa through the proper mucosal layer (Figure 5.4). The appearance of neoplasm blood vessels in sm cancer is roughly divided under two very characteristic observations. Although IPCL pattern V-3 (irregular vessels) is seen a lot in m3/sm1 cancer, it is observed near the superficial layer of the lesion under magnifying observation. On the other hand, IPCL pattern VN (new tumor vessels) is characteristic to sm deep invasive carcinoma (sm invasion depth is 200 μm and more), and is thicker than the blood vessel of IPCL pattern V-3 under magnifying observation, and is observed within the deep portion of the lesion (Figure 5.11).

DIFFERENCES SEEN FROM CAPILLARY PATTERNS (IPCL PATTERN CLASSIFICATION) BETWEEN "M1/M2" AND "CANCER THAT IS DEEPER THAN M3/SM1"

IPCL pattern classification of a superficial vessel is based on serial changes to the IPCL in normal epithelium. Therefore, changes that occur from IPCL Type II to Type V-2 take place within the mucosal layer keeping the original IPCL structure. The resulting changes to the IPCL exist within a vertical plane.

On the other hand, irregularly arranged IPCL in m3/sm1 involves the advance destruction of the original IPCL and runs in a horizontal plane (Figure 5.10(g)). It is recognized as running across abnormal blood vessels (Figure 5.10(h)). In IPCL Type VN, original IPCLs are totally destroyed, and a large-caliber new tumor vessel runs in a horizontal direction (Figure 5.11(e)).

IPCL Types V-1 and V-2 which often corresponds to m1/m2 lesion in histology, a changed IPCL still runs perpendicular. In IPCL Types V-3 and VN which closely relates to sm cancer in histology, IPCL runs in a horizontal direction.

The diagnostic difference between IPCL Types V-3 and VN is based upon the caliber of the new tumor vessels, and the histological depth where it appears. Tumor vessel which appears in IPCL Type VN is around 10 times larger than irregular vessel which appears in IPCL Type V-3.

We performed upper gastrointestinal endoscopy using magnifying endoscopy for 648 consecutive cases. Among them 250 cases received NBI magnifying endoscopy. The correct diagnosis ratio was 78%. All inconsistencies except one were in one category only.

One case of m1 lesion was over-estimation of submucosal invasive cancer during magnifying endoscopic survey. By reviewing the videotape, magnifying observation of previous biopsy scar looked like the finding of sm massive invasive cancer.

"PINK-SILVER SIGN" IN NBI OBSERVATION

Recognition of "pink color sign" in the non-iodine-stained lesions confirms the existence of carcinoma in situ or a deeper invasive lesion. "Pink color sign" is emphasized with NBI system and is recognized as "shiny silver sign" (Figures 5.10(c), (d) and 5.11(c), (d)). This is an additional useful finding for NBI observation. "Shiny silver sign" starts appearing around 7 minutes after iodine staining. This process will be shortened by spraying of sodium thiosulfate solution immediately after iodine staining. Combination of both phenonena is called "pink-silver sign".

THE ROUTE TO DETECT 1 MM CANCEROUS LESION

Recently, even the super-minute 1mm neoplasia can be detected. We have observed isolated 22 lesions out of 17 cases in the esophagus. You need to be careful not to overlook the minute lesion, which presents the same endoscopic findings as an intraepithelial spreading portion of esophageal submucosal invasive cancer. When the mucosa is observed under normal endoscopic observation, first attention needs to be paid to reddening areas. A novel developed NBI system allows us to detect this type of lesion as brown spot much easier (Figure 5.12). We suspected cancer when we found the following four conditions while performing magnifying endoscopic observation of a reddening spot white light or a brown spot in NBI enhanced image:

1 Area formation.

2 Loss of visibility of the green branching vessels in the lesion.

3 Marginal elevation of surrounding mucosa.

4 Change in vascular pattern to IPCL Types IV and V-1.

Whenever all of the above four factors being recognized, we strongly suspect carcinoma in situ (category IV of the Vienna classification).

Although the initial nine cases we detected the minute cancerous lesion through regular white light endoscopy, the remaining cases (majority of cases) were detected by observing brown spots under NBI observation. Through the emphasis of NBI imaging a detection of a minute cancer becomes easier.

CONCLUSIONS

In the pharynx and esophagus, which are covered with stratified squamous epithelium, NBI-magnified imaging allows us to observe IPCL micro-vascular structure well. IPCL pattern classification is corresponding well to histological changes in the squamous epithelium [see DVD video clips 9 and 10].

REFERENCES

1. Inoue H, Takeshita K, Hori H, et al. Endoscopic mucosal resection with a cap-fitted panendoscope for esophagus, stomach and colon mucosal lesions. *Gastrointest Endosc* 1993; 39: 58–62.
2. Ono H, Kondo H, Gotoda T, et al. Endoscopic mucosal resection for treatment of early gastric cancer. *Gut* 2001; 48: 225–229.
3. Inoue H. Treatment of esophageal and gastric tumors. *Endoscopy* 2001; 33: 119–125.
4. Endo M, Kawano T, Inoue H, et al. Clinicopathological analysis of lymph node metastasis in surgically resected superficial cancer of the thoracic esophagus. *Dis Esophagus* 2000; 13: 125–129.
5. Inoue H, Honda T, Yoshida T, et al. Ultra-high magnification endoscopy of the normal esophageal mucosa. *Dig Endosc* 1996; 8: 13–138.
6. Inoue H, Honda T, Nagai K, et al. Ultra-high magnification endoscopic observation of carcinoma in situ of the esophagus. *Dig Endosc* 1997; 9: 16–18.
7. Inoue H. Magnification endoscopy in the esophagus and stomach. *Dig Endosc* 2001; 13: 40–41.
8. Schlemper RJ, Riddell RH, Kato Y, et al. The Vienna classification of gastrointestinal epithelial neoplasia. *Gut* 2000; 47: 251–255.

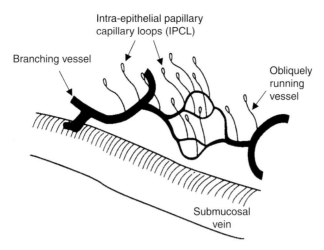

Intra-epithelial papillary
capillary loops (IPCL)

Branching vessel

Obliquely
running
vessel

Submucosal
vein

Figure 5.1 Schematic drawing of magnifying endoscopic findings for superficial blood vessels in the squamous esophagus. Superficial blood vessels in the esophageal mucosa consist of branching vessels which extend to the horizontal plane and exist immediately above the lamina muscularis mucosae. IPCL rises from a branching vessel perpendicularly. The blood vessel, which can be observed under regular non-magnifying endoscopy, is the branching vessel. When esophageal squmaous mucosa is magnified up to around 100 times through magnifying endoscopy, looping vessels (IPCL) are observed, as shown in Figure 5.2. IPCL is demonstrated as brown dots under NBI enhanced observation, as shown in Figure 5.5(b) (80-fold magnification). IPCL demonstrates characteristic changes in shape in carcinoma in situ (Figure 5.3). Through changes in the shape of the IPCL, the histological nature of the flat epithelial lesion and depth of cancer invasion can be possibly assessed (Copyright H. Inoue, M. Kaga, Y. Sato, S. Sugaya, S. Kudo).

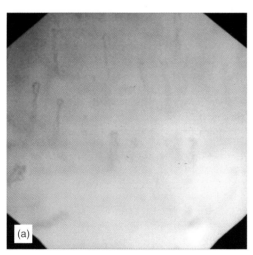

(a)

150X Prototype Olympus

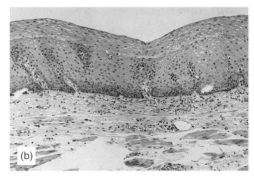

(b)

Figure 5.2 IPCL (intra-epithelial papillary capillary loop). (a) Magnified image of IPCL, using a prototype magnifying endoscope from Olympus with 150 times view. (b) Conventional histological image of normal mucosa in the esophagus. A part of *lamina propria mucosae* bulges up into stratified squamous epithelium as a papilla. This surface of papilla is covered with the epithelial basal layer. In this papilla, blood vessels of lamina propria mucosae rise in the shape of the papillary loop in the squamous epithelium, which is named the IPCL (Copyright H. Inoue, M. Kaga, Y. Sato, S. Sugaya, S. Kudo).

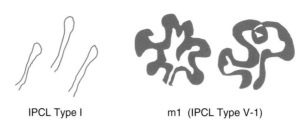

IPCL Type I   m1 (IPCL Type V-1)

Figure 5.3 In normal epithelium, IPCL is observed as a smooth running small-diameter capillary vessel (IPCL Type I). In carcinoma in situ IPCL demonstrates characteristic changes in its figure. The abnormal IPCL pattern for m1 lesion (carcinoma in situ) becomes IPCL Type V-1, which shows the following four patterns; dilation, meandering, irregular caliber, and form variation (Copyright H. Inoue, M. Kaga, Y. Sato, S. Sugaya, S. Kudo).

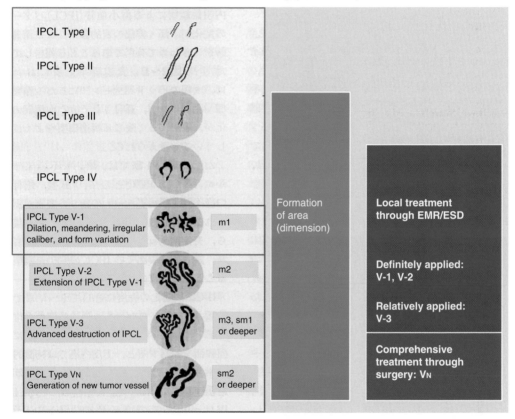

Figure 5.4 IPCL pattern classification includes two sets of diagnostic criteria. IPCL pattern classification from IPCL Type I to Type V-1 demonstrates the tissue characterization for flat lesion (square with red line). IPCL pattern classification from IPCL Type V-1 to Type VN reflects cancer infiltration depth (square with blue line). IPCL Type III corresponds to borderline lesion which potentially includes esophagitis, low-grade intraepithelial neoplasia. IPCL Type III should be considered for a further follow-up study. In IPCL Type IV, high-grade intraepithelial neoplasia or carcinoma in situ appears, and then further treatment with EMR/ESD should be considered. EMR/ESD should be also considered for IPCL Types V-1 and V-2 as they are definite m1 or m2 lesion with no risk of lymph node metastasis. To IPCL Type V-3 lesion which corresponds to m3 lesion, diagnostic EMR/ESD should be applied as a complete biopsy to decide treatment strategy. Furthermore, IPCL Type VN corresponds to a new tumor vessel, which is the cancer often associated with sm2 invasion with significantly increasing risk of lymph node metastasis, and the surgical treatment should be recommended (Copyright H. Inoue, M. Kaga, Y. Sato, S. Sugaya, S. Kudo).

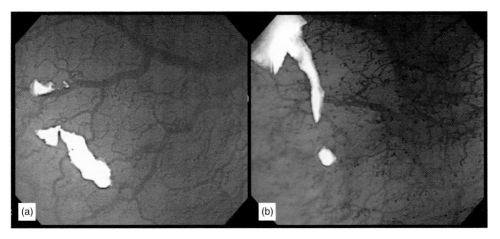

Figure 5.5 The IPCL image of normal mucosa (IPCL Type I). A commercially available high-definition magnifying endoscope has 80-fold magnification power and it allows us to observe IPCL pattern clearly particularly with NBI enhanced imaging (LUCERA system, optical zoom). (a) Magnifying observation under normal white light. The IPCL is a capillary vessel positioned upright from a branching vessel and is observed as a red dot in 80-fold magnification. (b) Magnification with NBI enhancement. Branching vessels which are located at the surface of *muscularis mucosae* are shown as a green vascular network expanding horizontally. The IPCL is observed as a brown vessel which is positioned in the most superficial layer and is derived upright from the branching vessel. Brownish IPCL has a high contrast to greenish branching vessel (Copyright H. Inoue, M. Kaga, Y. Sato, S. Sugaya, S. Kudo).

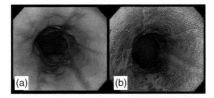

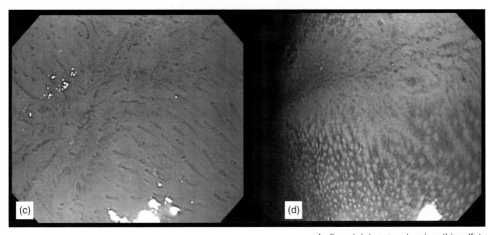

Iodine staining + potassium thiosulfate

Figure 5.6 IPCL Type II is often observed in gastroesophageal reflux disease. (a) Regular endoscopic image. GERD Los Angeles classification D. (b) Iodine staining delineates clearly the erosive mucosa. (c) IPCL extension (engorgement) is observed in GERD cases with magnifying endoscopy. In addition to this fact, the IPCL runs in the same direction. Although an irregular running is found in the central erosive part, the level of extension and meandering in IPCL is still limited to be mild change and the lesion margin is less clear and demarcated than that of neoplastic cases. (d) In magnifying endoscopy the lesion margin is demonstrated unclear under iodine staining (Copyright H. Inoue, M. Kaga, Y. Sato, S. Sugaya, S. Kudo).

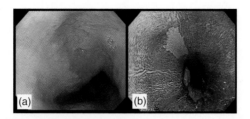

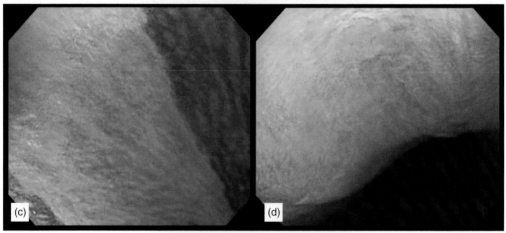

Iodine staining + potassium
thiosulfate

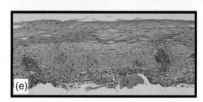

Figure 5.7 Chronic esophagitis (IPCL Type III). Although clear regional formation in non-iodine-stained area is recognized, no change of IPCL can be seen in the same area. That means no proliferation of tumorous vessels. (a) Regular endoscopy. Close-up view. Redness on mucosal surface was observed. (b) The lesion was demonstrated as iodine voiding area under iodine staining. (c) Close-up view of iodine voiding area. (d) Magnifying endoscopic view of the same area. No vessel proliferation was observed. The lesion was treated first by iodine and then by sodium thiosulfate. (e) Biopsy specimen from the non-iodine-stained area was histologically diagnosed as esophagitis (Copyright H. Inoue, M. Kaga, Y. Sato, S. Sugaya, S. Kudo).

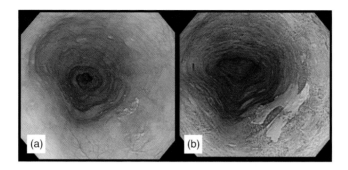

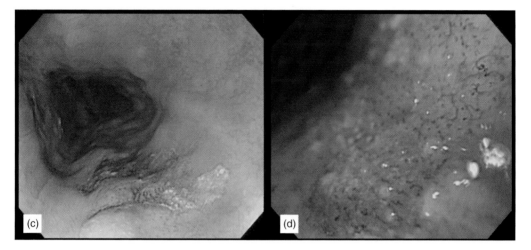

Figure 5.8 A lesion of IPCL Type IV. (a) Flat and small erosion is observed on the surface mucosa. (b) With iodine staining, it is shown as an iodine-void area with a well-defined boundary. (c) Under NBI imaging the lesion is shown as a brown spot. The brown spot is the combined image of both increased number of IPCL and brownish coloration in the background mucosa. (d) Although proliferation of blood vessels in the region is found, there is not so severe change as with IPCL Type V-1. Then we diagnosed it as IPCL Type IV.

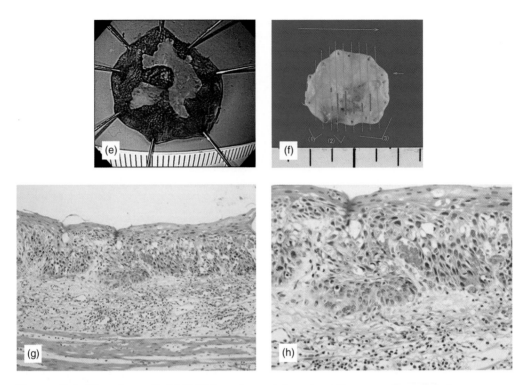

Figure 5.8 (Continued) (e) EMR is performed. Lugol-voiding area was resected as one-piece specimen. (f) The red lines indicate distribution of m1 cancer. IPCL Type IV often includes high-grade dysplasia and m1 cancer like in this case. (g and h) Histology of the lesion. It is diagnosed as non-invasive high-grade neoplasia (Copyright H. Inoue, M. Kaga, Y. Sato, S. Sugaya, S. Kudo).

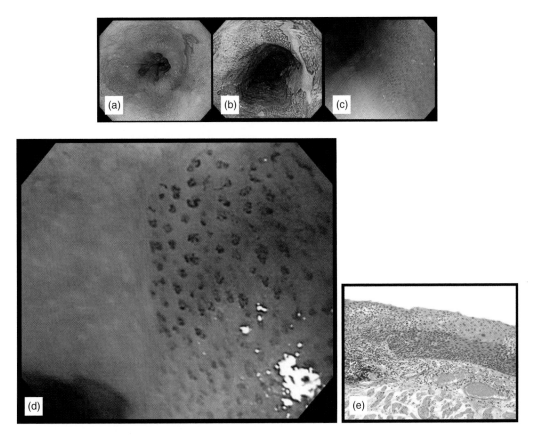

Figure 5.9 Typical image of IPCL Type V-1. (a) The lesion is observed as IIc (slightly depressed) with redness. (b) Under iodine staining, the lesion is observed as an iodine-voiding area, which corresponds to the red portion in Figure 5.9(a). (c) Under magnifying endoscopy, the color tone of red IIc lesion is shown as the synthesis of redness of enlarged IPCL and redness of the background mucosa. (d) This is a typical image of IPCL Type V-1 under magnifying endoscopy with NBI. The lesion is definitely diagnosed as m1. (e) Histopathological diagnosis on the ESD sample is m1 (Copyright H. Inoue, M. Kaga, Y. Sato, S. Sugaya, S. Kudo).

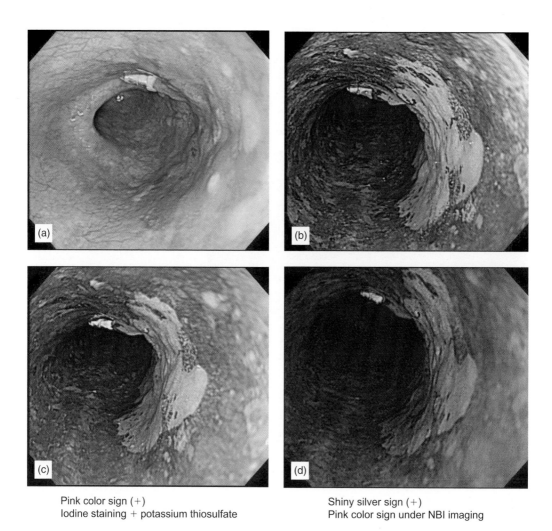

Pink color sign (+)
Iodine staining + potassium thiosulfate

Shiny silver sign (+)
Pink color sign under NBI imaging

Figure 5.10 0-IIc (IPCL Types V-1 to V-3). (a) Erosion can be seen in the normal image. The clip is only for hemostasis after biopsy and thus it does not have any diagnostic importance. This is a 0-IIc lesion extending from 1 to 5 o'clock, whose center shows short nodal uplift, and exceeds m2. However, there is no hard nodule which would suggest sm2 infiltration, so we diagnosed m3/sm1 infiltration in non-magnified endoscopic image. (b) Iodine staining. Cancerous lesion was clearly delineated. More insufflations are performed with iodine stain than with normal endoscopy (a). (c) Pink color sign and (d) shiny silver sign. In a couple of minutes after iodine staining, the cancer in the un-dyed area becomes pink, which is called "pink color sign". In non-cancerous lesions including LGD that fail to stain with Lugol's, such a transition over time from yellow to pink in the un-dyed area is not observed. In order to observe this change as soon as possible, it is better to spray sodium thiosulfate, and when the pink color sign looks observed with NBI, the area appears shiny silver. This is called "shiny silver sign". Combination of both phenomena is called "pink-silver sign."

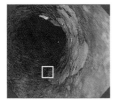

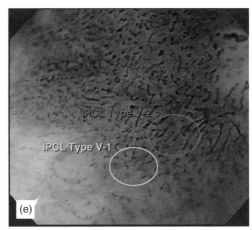

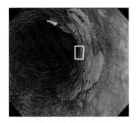

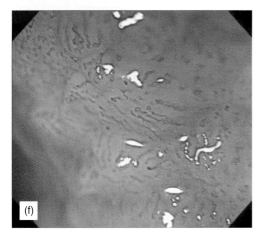

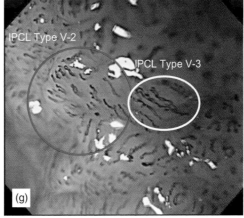

Figure 5.10 (Continued) Magnified endoscopic image. Enlarging the area in the white frame. (e) The change of IPCL Type V-1 is observed in the marginal regions (circled in yellow) and it is corresponding to m1 invasion depth. The change of IPCL Type V-2 is observed proximal to the margins and can be considered as m2 (circled in green). Most lesions of this type occur this way, with m1 and m2 classifications in one lesion. (f) and (g) With the center of the lesion (enlarged part in the white frame), IPCL Types V-2 and V-3 are observed (circled in green and white, respectively). Observe closely the comparison between normal magnification (f) and magnification with NBI (g). These two images are captured almost at the same position, but the NBI image has better contrast than the normal white light image. IPCL Type V-3 regarded as m3/sm1 invasion depth can be observed when the deeper IPCL with those four characteristics described in Figure 5.3 are observed and linked with each other in deeper layer.

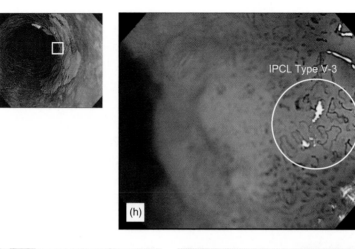

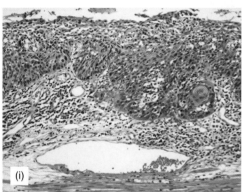

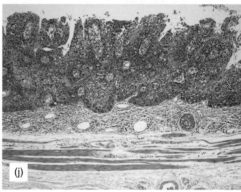

IPCL Type V-1   IPCL Type V-2

Figure 5.10 (Continued) (h) IPCL Type V-3. When the portion in the white frame is enlarged, transversely running and irregular-shaped blood vessels as IPCL deformation is found. The pattern of the vessel is categorized as IPCL Type V-3. (i) Histopathological image. In the marginal lesion recognized as IPCL Type V-1, infiltration is as deep as m1. Proximal to the margins, infiltration is m2 level. This histological part is corresponding with Figure 5.10(e). (j) Histopathological image. Most of the lesion is infiltrated as deeply as m2, but there are some areas with cancer invasion of the lamina propria mucosae, which extends very close to lamina muscularis mucosae. Pathology shows it is still m2 in most of the lesion, but it may well be diagnosed as m3 in a demonstrated image (Copyright H. Inoue, M. Kaga, Y. Sato, S. Sugaya, S. Kudo).

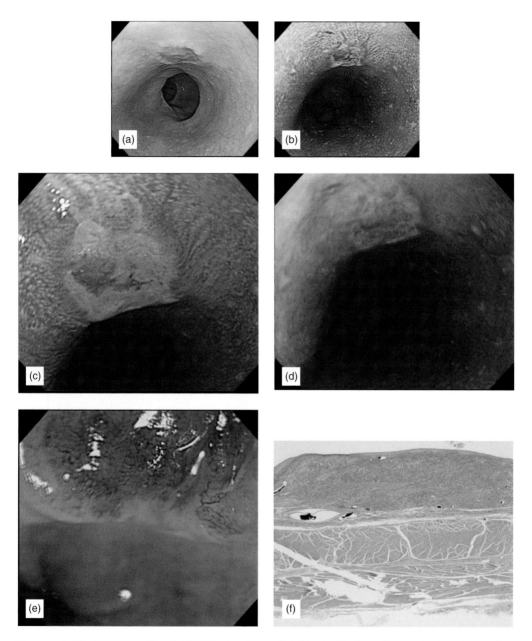

Figure 5.11 IPCL Type Vn. (a) 0-III lesion (superficial but with deep depression) is observed with normal endoscopy, sm invasive cancer is suspected because of central concavity with marginal uplift. (b) Area with cancer exposure was sharply demonstrated. The exterior of marginal uplift is dyed with iodine. Regenerating epithelium dyed by iodine is also observed in the area of concavity due to previous biopsy. (c) Close image with iodine stain. A couple of minutes after iodine stain. The exposed tumor shows "pink color sign". (d) NBI image in a couple of minutes after iodine stain. The exposed tumor shows "shiny silver sign" which corresponds to "pink color sign" in white light. Both phenomena (c) and (d) are called "pink-silver sign". (e) Magnified NBI image after iodine stain. New tumor vessel with large diameter (Vn: new tumor vessel) is observed. Vn is usually transversely oriented. The lesion can be diagnosed as sm massive cancer if such Vn is widely found in the lesion. (f) Histopathological image. Squamous cancer, sm2 invasion (Copyright H. Inoue, M. Kaga, Y. Sato, S. Sugaya, S. Kudo).

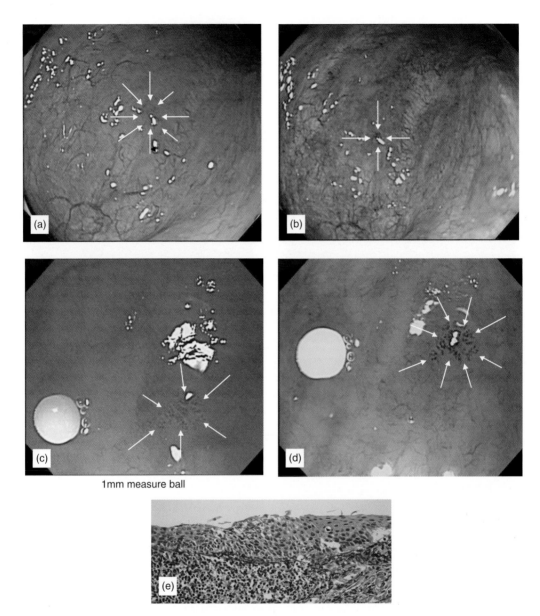

1mm measure ball

Figure 5.12 1 mm cancerous lesion at the posterior of pharynx. (a) The lesion is observed only as a small point of redness in close image under normal endoscopy. (b) The lesion is recognized as a brown spot by NBI (white arrows). It is important not to overlook such a small red point (i.e. blown spot in NBI) while inserting the endoscope. (c) An image with magnifying endoscopy. The white ball which is attached closely to the lesion has 1 mm outer diameter. The lesion indicated with white arrows is 1 mm in size. (d) Magnified image with NBI enhancement. It is categorized as a lesion of IPCL Type IV with its own range. (e) Histological analysis for a sample of biopsy. Squamous cell cancer. If the lesion is no more than 1 mm wide, the treatment is completed even with bite biopsy (Copyright H. Inoue, M. Kaga, Y. Sato, S. Sugaya, S. Kudo).

Applications of NBI HRE and preliminary data: Barrett's esophagus and adenocarcinoma

6

Wouter Curvers, Paul Fockens and Jacques Bergman

INTRODUCTION

Esophageal adenocarcinoma and Barrett's esophagus

Esophageal adenocarcinoma is the cancer with the most rapidly rising incidence in the Western World and has a known precursor lesion called Barrett's esophagus (BE) [1] (Figure 6.1). BE is a complication of chronic gastro-esophageal reflux, in which the normal stratified squamous epithelium of the distal esophagus has been replaced by columnar epithelium with specialized intestinal metaplasia (IM) (Figure 6.2). To meet the current definition of BE, endoscopic evidence of a columnar-lined distal esophagus and histological evidence of IM are required [2,3].

Although the exact mechanisms of carcinogenesis are not fully understood, experts believe that malignant transformation in BE involves a metaplasia–dysplasia–carcinoma sequence [4]. In this process, low-grade dysplasia (LGD), high-grade dysplasia (HGD) and early (mucosal) cancer (EC) may precede the development of invasive cancer [5]. The continuous rise in incidence and the poor prognosis associated with esophageal adenocarcinoma have driven research into finding ways of early detection of neoplastic changes in BE.

Current recommendations are to offer patients with BE regular endoscopic surveillance in order to detect those early lesions in an early and curable stage [2,3]. The effectiveness of these guidelines, however, is hampered by several factors including the subtleness of early neoplastic lesions making their detection with standard endoscopic techniques difficult (Figure 6.3). When no abnormalities are detected during endoscopy, which is the case in most patients, the diagnosis of any neoplasia relies on randomly acquired biopsy samples. However, even the most rigorous random biopsy protocol is associated with sampling error and therefore an inevitable miss rate [6].

In order to improve the detection rate of neoplasia and the efficacy of endoscopic surveillance endoscopy in BE patients, various advanced endoscopic imaging modalities have recently been investigated.

High-resolution magnification endoscopy and chromoendoscopy

Magnification endoscopes, equipped with high-quality charge coupled devices and an adjustable focal length, allow for detailed inspection of the superficial mucosal and vascular patterns (i.e. "mucosal morphology"). Magnifying endoscopy has been shown to improve the detection of specialized IM (and to a lesser extent of early neoplasia) in BE. This is usually achieved by combining magnification endoscopy with chromoendoscopy [7].

Chromoendoscopy is a technique in which dyes are sprayed on the mucosal surface in order to enhance the detection and/ or delineation of early neoplastic lesions. Some studies have shown that chromoendoscopy may improve the detection of neoplasia but others have failed to confirm these findings [8–11]. In addition this technique is associated with some important limitations. First, it requires the use of dyes and spraying catheters and lengthens the total procedure time. Second, the technique is operator dependent and requires experience for optimal results. Third, dye may not spread evenly across the mucosa. Fourth, switching between the white light view and the enhanced pattern chromoendoscopy view is impossible. Finally, the mucosal morphology consists of both the mucosal and the vascular patterns of which the latter may be obscured by the use of stains.

Several classification systems for the mucosal patterns in BE have been proposed using chromoendoscopy [8,12,13]. Most of these studies, however, concentrated on differentiating normal gastric-type mucosal patterns from intestinal-type mucosal patterns, while mucosal pattern appearance of early neoplasia has more clinical relevance. All proposed classifications depend on detecting minute differences in the size and shape of the mucosal pits and ridges, which may make inter-observer agreement difficult.

Narrowband imaging

Narrow band imaging (NBI) is a novel endoscopic imaging technique which may enhance the mucosal surface contrast without the use of dyes. NBI makes use of the optical phenomenon that the depth of light penetration into tissues is dependent on the wavelength; the shorter the wavelength the more super-ficial the penetration. Therefore, in the visible spectrum, blue light penetrates most superficially (i.e. mucosal imaging) while red light penetrates the deepest (i.e. submucosal imaging). In addition, short wavelength light also causes less scattering. In NBI, the band-pass ranges of the red, green and blue components of white light have been narrowed and the relative intensity of blue light has been increased.

MUCOSAL MORPHOLOGY OF BE USING NBI

Since the development of the prototype NBI system, several studies have indicated that this technique elegantly displays the mucosal and vascular patterns in different organ systems [14–16]. A number of reports have indicated that NBI may also be helpful in revealing suspicious areas in BE [17]. In this regard, it has been postulated that NBI may lead to the same contrast enhancement capabilities as chromoendoscopy but without its aforementioned disadvantages.

In order to investigate the mucosal morphology characteristics of early neoplasia and non-dysplastic mucosa we investigated 63 BE patients (including 41 with HGD/EC) with high-resolution white light endoscopy and NBI [18]. Magnified images and corresponding biopsies were taken and evaluated blindly. The data was randomly dived into an explorative set, a learning set and a validation set.

Explorative phase

In the explorative phase, images and biopsies of 15 areas were reviewed by the study's expert pathologist and two endo-scopists in an unblinded manner. Insight gained from this exploratory meeting and from previously published classifi-cations using chromoendoscopy was used to develop stand-ardized forms of both image and bio evaluation. During the exploratory evaluation, it was observed that the mucosal mor-phology consisted of mucosal patterns (in accordance with the literature) but also vascular patterns were observed, which were not previously described. Therefore all images were eval-uated during the following two phases (learning and validation phase) for: (1) the type of mucosal pattern (flat mucosa, circular/oval/tubular pattern, longitudinal pattern, villous/gyrus-like pattern and disrupted mucosa), (2) the regularity of the mucosal pattern (regular, focally irregular/disrupted, diffusely irregular/disrupted), (3) the presence of a vascular pattern, (4) the regular-ity of the vascular pattern (regular, focally irregular or diffusely irregular), (5) whether the vasculature formed honeycomb structures, (6) whether all blood vessels were situated between or alongside the mucosal folds, (7) the presence of blood vessels crossing over mucosal folds ("mucosal bridging"), (8) in the case of a flat mucosa, whether the vasculature consisted of normal-appearing long-branching vessels, (9) the presence of abnormal blood vessels and (10) description of the observed abnormal vessels.

Prior to the study, the protocol required the evaluation of both white light and NBI images. But during early endoscopic evaluation and the exploratory meeting it became obvious that the NBI images were clearly superior for detailed inspection of the mucosal morphology. Therefore white light images were excluded from subsequent analysis.

Learning phase

Non-dysplatic BE

Of the 52 evaluated areas, 24 were found to contain non-dysplastic BE. Nineteen (79%) showed villous/gyrus-forming mucosal patterns on the NBI images and 5 areas (21%) showed flat mucosa without evidence of pit patterns or mucosal folds. Of the 19 areas with villous/gyrus-forming patterns, 12 (63%) were evaluated as having regular mucosal patterns.

The vascular pattern was recognized in 23 areas (96%). A regular vascular pattern was found in 17 (89%) of the 19 areas with a villous/gyrus-forming mucosal pattern with all of the blood vessels regularly situated between or along the mucosal folds. All of the 5 areas with a flat mucosa showed a regular pattern with normal-appearing long-branching blood vessels.

Figure 6.4 shows typical examples of the regular villous patterns (Figure 6.4(a)–(d)) and flat mucosa with long-branching blood vessels (Figure 6.4(e) and (f)) which were found to be the main characteristics of non-dysplastic IM.

Early neoplasia

There were 14 areas with HGD/EC in the learning set. Eleven areas (79%) showed irregular/disrupted mucosal patterns. The mucosal patterns were judged to be villous/gyrus-forming in 10 areas. Of the 14 areas with HGD/EC, the vascular pattern was recognized in 12 (86%); of these 12 areas, the vascular pattern was scored as irregular in 9 (75%). Abnormal blood vessels were found in 9 areas (75%); in 8 of the 9 cases (89%) there was more than one abnormality; spiral vessels, caliber changes and small isolated vessels being the most common abnormalities. Figure 6.5 shows an example of irregular mucosal and vascular patterns (Figure 6.5(a)–(d)) and abnormal blood vessels (Figure 6.5(e) and (f)).

Relevant factors

When comparing the mucosal morphology features of the non-dysplastic BE areas with the rest of the learning set, the regular villous/gyrus-forming mucosal pattern was significantly associated with non-dysplastic BE ($p = 0.009$). In addition, the flat-type mucosa with long-branching normal-appearing vessels was 100% (5/5) associated with non-dysplastic IM. No other image variable was found to be significantly associated with non-dysplastic IM. On the other hand, the irregular/disrupted mucosal pattern was found to be significantly associated with HGD ($p = 0.03$). The presence of abnormal blood vessels was also significantly associated with HGD/EC ($p < 0.001$). No other image variable was found to be significantly associated with HGD/EC.

Validation phase

For both non-dysplastic BE and HGD/EC, the results of the learning set were reproduced in the validation set. Of the 55 areas with non-dysplastic BE, 45 (82%) showed villous/gyrus-forming mucosal patterns with regular vascular patterns in 40 areas. Ten areas (18%) showed flat mucosa, 8 with regular long-branching normal-appearing blood vessels.

Of the 34 areas with HGD/EC, 32 (94%) showed irregular/disrupted mucosal patterns, all of which were judged to be of the villous/gyrus-forming type. The vasculature was recognized in 31 areas; the vascular pattern was scored as irregular in 29 (94%). Abnormal blood vessels were found in 27 areas (87%); in 20 of the 27 cases (74%) there was more than one abnormality. The most common abnormalities in the blood vessels were again spiral vessels, caliber changes and small isolated vessels.

The flat-type mucosa ($p = 0.01$) and the regular villous/gyrus-forming mucosal pattern ($p = 0.02$) were found to be independent predictors of the presence of non-dysplastic BE and (1) an irregular/disrupted mucosal pattern ($p = 0.03$), (2) an irregular vascular pattern ($p = 0.004$), and (3) the presence of abnormal blood vessels ($p = 0.005$) were found to be independent predictors for HGD/EC.

In addition, all areas with HGD/EC were found to have at least one of the following three characteristics: (1) an irregular/disrupted mucosal pattern, (2) an irregular vascular pattern or (3) abnormal blood vessels. Twenty-nine of the 34 areas with HGD/EC (85%) had two or more of these characteristics.

Three-step classification system of mucosal morphology

Based on these results, a three-step classification system was developed for the mucosal morphology in BE (Table 6.1). This

Regularity mucosal pattern	Regular	Irregular
Regularity vascular pattern	Regular	Irregular
Presence of abnormal blood vessels	Not present	Present

Table 6.1 Hierarchical three-step classification system for mucosal morphology in BE.

classification system was used with the aforementioned data. All areas with regular mucosal/vascular patterns without abnormal blood vessels as well as areas with a flat mucosa and no abnormal blood vessels were considered "*not suspicious*" for dysplasia. Areas were considered "*suspicious*" for dysplasia/ cancer if they had at least one of the following three characteristics: (1) irregular/disrupted mucosal pattern, (2) irregular vascular pattern (3) and/or abnormal blood vessels. Using this risk-stratification model, a sensitivity of 100% and a specificity of 61% were obtained for HGD/EC.

Based on these results, we postulated that detection of the mucosal pattern should be followed by determination of its regularity/irregularity since irregular patterns may be associated with a higher chance of dysplasia/cancer. The next step is the detection of the vascular pattern and determination of its regularity/irregularity since it forms an integral and clinically relevant part of the mucosal morphology. Subsequently, the mucosa should be evaluated for the presence of abnormal blood vessels since their presence is one of the three abnormalities that may raise a suspicion for dysplasia/cancer.

DETECTING EARLY NEOPLASIA IN BE USING NBI

Sharma et al. found that the detection of neoplastic lesions may be improved by looking at the mucosal patterns in BE using indigo carmine chromoendoscopy (ICC) [8]. After we evaluated which NBI characteristics are relevant to discriminate non-dysplastic BE from early neoplasia, we performed a clinical study comparing NBI with ICC in a randomized cross-over design [19].

Twenty-eight patients with BE referred for the work-up of endoscopically inconspicuous early neoplasia underwent high-resolution endoscopy (HRE) plus NBI and HRE plus ICC in a randomized cross-over design separated by an interval of 6–8 weeks. The two procedures were performed by two different endoscopists, who were blinded to the findings of the other examination. Targeted biopsies were taken from all detected lesions followed by 2-cm-interval-4-quadrant biopsies. Histopathological evaluation was supervised by a single expert pathologist who was blinded to the imaging technique used. In total, 14 patients were diagnosed with HGD/EC. The per patient sensitivity for HGD/EC was 93% for HRE plus NBI and 86% for HRE plus ICC (Figure 6.6), with targeted biopsies using both techniques diagnosing 79% of patients with HGD/EC. More importantly, all patients detected by targeted biopsies were already diagnosed using HRE only. ICC detected four additional lesions of which two contained HGD/EC and NBI detected nine additional lesions, four of which contained HGD/EC. These lesions, however, did not alter the sensitivity for identifying patients with HGD/EC.

Although ICC and NBI did not improve the detection of HGD/EC, this study has shown that NBI is at least as good as ICC for imaging Barrett mucosa. As highlighted above, NBI has a number of advantages over chromoendoscopy. First, it is user friendly with its application only requiring a touch of a button. There is no need for dyes, spraying catheters or extensive washouts and aspirations. Second, the epithelial (micro) vascular patterns are better viewed with NBI than with chromoendoscopy. In particular, the vascular bed in the areas between the mucosal folds can be observed with NBI but not with chromoendoscopy, since the dye accumulates in these grooves. In contrast, NBI does not require any specific skills. Moreover, the technique of NBI is relatively simple and incurs no extra per case costs associated with dye and spray catheters.

A potential problem with NBI is observer variation in the interpretation of the images. However, this holds for chromoendoscopy too. There is no data yet to address the question of the length of the learning curve before endoscopists can reliably detect the characteristic patterns of HGD/EC using NBI HRE.

The failure of these techniques to improve the sensitivity for HGD/EC in BE when compared to HRE alone in this study can be at least partly explained by the fact that these techniques are most suitable in BE for *targeted inspection* of areas of interest and less suitable for *primary detection* of abnormalities. This limitation is inherent in both techniques because their objective is to reveal the details of the (micro) structures present on the mucosal surface. To achieve this objective, magnification and therefore targeted inspection of a small area is necessary. Hence, ideally, suspicious areas should be detected first before applying either ICC or NBI since the power of these techniques lies in detailed inspection of focal lesions.

In this perspective NBI could serve as an adjunct to autofluorescence video endoscopy. Autofluorescence video endoscopy is an advanced imaging technique that may improve the detection of early neoplasia. In autofluorescence, certain endogenous molecules emit fluorescence light when they are excited with short wavelength light (e.g. blue light). It has been shown with endoscopic point spectroscopy that early neoplasia in BE can be distinguished from non-dysplastic BE based on differences in autofluorescence and reflectance spectra [20]. In autofluorescence video endoscopy this technique is used in a real-time wide-angle endoscopy system. In a recent feasibility study we showed that one of the drawbacks of this technique is the high percentage of false positive lesions that were detected with autofluorescence video endoscopy [21].

NBI can be used for a subsequent characterization of suspicious areas detected with autofluorescence video endoscopy. In a proof-of-principle study, we examined 20 BE patients with suspected or endoscopically treated early neoplasia using two separate imaging systems: autofluorescence video endoscopy and NBI [22]. Of the 28 lesions with early neoplasia, 17 were identified with HRE (61%) and 28 with autofluorescence video endoscopy (100%). Forty-seven suspicious lesions were detected with autofluorescence video endoscopy: 28 contained early neoplasia: 19 were false positive (40%). With NBI, suspicious patterns were found in all lesions with early neoplasia, while regular patterns were found in 14 of the 19 false positive lesions. The false positive rate was therefore reduced to 10% and of the 5 remaining false positive lesions, 4 contained LGD (Figure 6.7). This proof-of-principle study shows that NBI may be used for *targeted inspection* to verify the surface pattern characteristics of suspicious lesions detected with an overview imaging technique, such as autofluorescence video endoscopy. Recently a new endoscopic system has been developed that incorporates HRE, autofluorescence video endoscopy and NBI [23] [see DVD video clips 11–14].

CONCLUSION

NBI is a promising new technique that may have additional value for imaging BE and the management of patients with early BE neoplasia.

It is a relatively simple and easy technique that has the advantages of chromoendoscopy but does not require the use of staining agents.

In addition, NBI reveals additional features of the mucosal morphology (i.e. blood vessels) that are not easily recognized with high-resolution magnification endoscopy and chromoendoscopy. These features may help to distinguish non-dysplastic BE from neoplastic areas.

In BE, NBI appears to be the most suited for targeted inspection of areas of interest after primary detection of these areas, either with HRE or other "red-flag" techniques under development.

REFERENCES

1. Devesa SS, Blot WJ, Fraumeni JF Jr. Changing patterns in the incidence of esophageal and gastric carcinoma in the United States. *Cancer* 1998; 83(10): 2049–2053.
2. Hirota WK, Zuckerman MJ, Adler DG, Davila RE, Egan J, Leighton JA, et al. ASGE guideline: the role of endoscopy in the surveillance of premalignant conditions of the upper GI tract. *Gastrointest Endosc* 2006; 63(4): 570–580.
3. Sampliner RE. Updated guidelines for the diagnosis, surveillance, and therapy of Barrett's esophagus. *Am J Gastroenterol* 2002; 97(8): 1888–1895.
4. Tytgat GN, Hameeteman W, Onstenk R, Schotborg R. The spectrum of columnar-lined esophagus – Barrett's esophagus. *Endoscopy* 1989; 21(4): 177–185.
5. Hameeteman W, Tytgat GN, Houthoff HJ, van den Tweel JG. Barrett's esophagus: development of dysplasia and adenocarcinoma. *Gastroenterology* 1989; 96(5 Pt 1): 1249–1256.
6. Falk GW, Rice TW, Goldblum JR, Richter JE. Jumbo biopsy forceps protocol still misses unsuspected cancer in Barrett's esophagus with high-grade dysplasia. *Gastrointest Endosc* 1999; 49(2): 170–176.
7. Bruno MJ. Magnification endoscopy, high resolution endoscopy, and chromoscopy; towards a better optical diagnosis. *Gut* 2003; 52(Suppl. 4): iv7–iv11.
8. Sharma P, Weston AP, Topalovski M, Cherian R, Bhattacharyya A, Sampliner RE. Magnification chromoendoscopy for the detection of intestinal metaplasia and dysplasia in Barrett's oesophagus. *Gut* 2003; 52(1): 24–27.
9. Egger K, Werner M, Meining A, Ott R, Allescher HD, Hofler H, et al. Biopsy surveillance is still necessary in patients with Barrett's oesophagus despite new endoscopic imaging techniques. *Gut* 2003; 52(1): 18–23.
10. Hoffman A, Kiesslich R, Bender A, Neurath MF, Nafe B, Herrmann G, et al. Acetic acid-guided biopsies after magnifying endoscopy compared with random biopsies in the detection of Barrett's esophagus: a prospective randomized trial with crossover design. *Gastrointest Endosc* 2006; 64(1): 1–8.
11. Ferguson DD, DeVault KR, Krishna M, Loeb DS, Wolfsen HC, Wallace MB. Enhanced magnification-directed biopsies do not increase the detection of intestinal metaplasia in patients with GERD. *Am J Gastroenterol* 2006; 101(7): 1611–1616.
12. Guelrud M, Ehrlich EE. Endoscopic classification of Barrett's esophagus. *Gastrointest Endosc* 2004; 59(1): 58–65.
13. Endo T, Awakawa T, Takahashi H, Arimura Y, Itoh F, Yamashita K, et al. Classification of Barrett's epithelium by magnifying endoscopy. *Gastrointest Endosc* 2002; 55(6): 641–647.
14. Hamamoto Y, Endo T, Nosho K, Arimura Y, Sato M, Imai K. Usefulness of narrow-band imaging endoscopy for diagnosis of Barrett's esophagus. *J Gastroenterol* 2004; 39(1): 14–20.
15. Yoshida T, Inoue H, Usui S, Satodate H, Fukami N, Kudo SE. Narrow-band imaging system with magnifying endoscopy for superficial esophageal lesions. *Gastrointest Endosc* 2004; 59(2): 288–295.

16. Machida H, Sano Y, Hamamoto Y, Muto M, Kozu T, Tajiri H, et al. Narrow-band imaging in the diagnosis of colorectal mucosal lesions: a pilot study. *Endoscopy* 2004; 36(12): 1094–1098.
17. Sharma P, Bansal A, Mathur S, Wani S, Cherian R, McGregor D, et al. The utility of a novel narrow band imaging endoscopy system in patients with Barrett's esophagus. *Gastrointest Endosc* 2006; 64(2): 167–175.
18. Kara MA, Ennahachi M, Fockens P, ten Kate FJ, Bergman JJ. Detection and classification of the mucosal and vascular patterns (mucosal morphology) in Barrett's esophagus by using narrow band imaging. *Gastrointest Endosc* 2006; 64(2): 155–166.
19. Kara MA, Peters FP, Rosmolen WD, Krishnadath KK, ten Kate FJ, Fockens P, et al. High-resolution endoscopy plus chromoendoscopy or narrow-band imaging in Barrett's esophagus: a prospective randomized crossover study. *Endoscopy* 2005; 37(10): 929–936.
20. Georgakoudi I, Jacobson BC, Van Dam J, Backman V, Wallace MB, Muller MG, et al. Fluorescence, reflectance, and light-scattering spectroscopy for evaluating dysplasia in patients with Barrett's esophagus. *Gastroenterology* 2001; 120(7): 1620–1629.
21. Kara MA, Peters FP, ten Kate FJW, van Deventer SJ, Fockens P, Bergman JJGHM. Endoscopic video autofluorescence imaging may improve the detection of early neoplasia in patients with Barrett's esophagus. *Gastrointest Endosc* 2005; 61(6): 679–685.
22. Kara MA, Peters FP, Fockens P, ten Kate FJ, Bergman JJ. Endoscopic video-autofluorescence imaging followed by narrow band imaging for detecting early neoplasia in Barrett's esophagus. *Gastrointest Endosc* 2006; 64(2): 176–185.
23. Curvers WL, Wong Kee Song LM, Wang K, Gostout CJ, Wallace MB, Wolfsen HC, et al. Endoscopic tri-modal imaging (ETMI) for the detection of dysplastic lesions in Barrett's esophagus. *Gastroenterology* 2006; 130(4 Suppl. 2): A642.

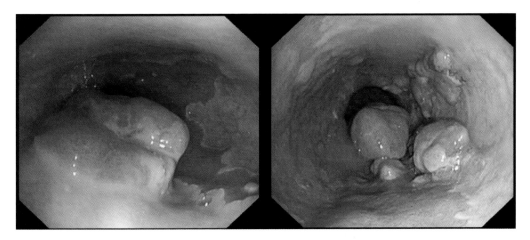

Figure 6.1 Esophageal adenocarcinoma.

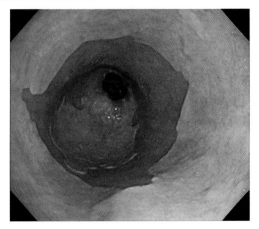

Figure 6.2 Barrett's esophagus.

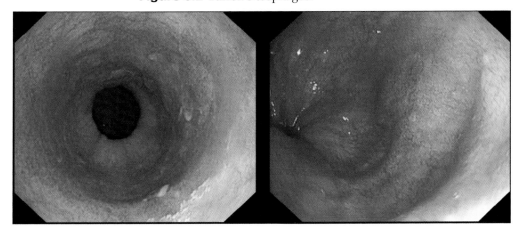

Figure 6.3 Two images with discrete early neoplastic lesions in a BE at the 3 o'clock position.

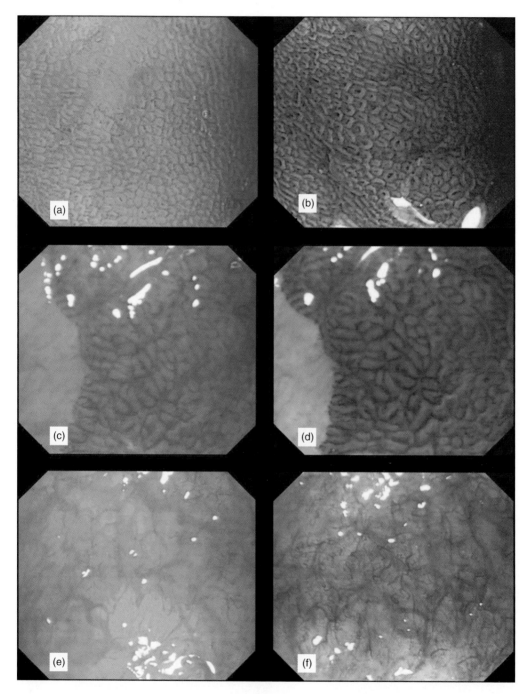

Figure 6.4 Examples of regular mucosal and vascular patterns of the villous/gyrus type ((a)–(d)) and flat mucosa with long-branching blood vessels ((e) and (f)). All these images contain non-dysplastic BE.

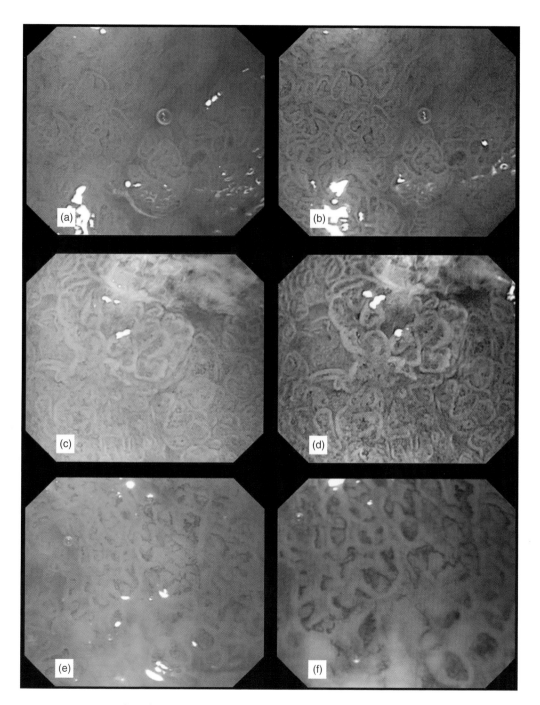

Figure 6.5 Examples of dysplastic BE with irregular and distorted mucosal and vascular patterns ((a)–(d)) and abnormal blood vessels ((e) and (f)).

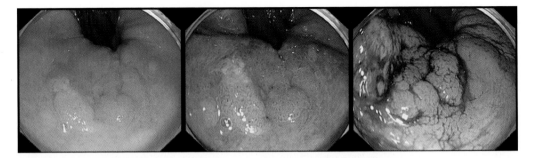

Figure 6.6 Imaging of an early neoplastic lesion in a BE using HRE, NBI and ICC.

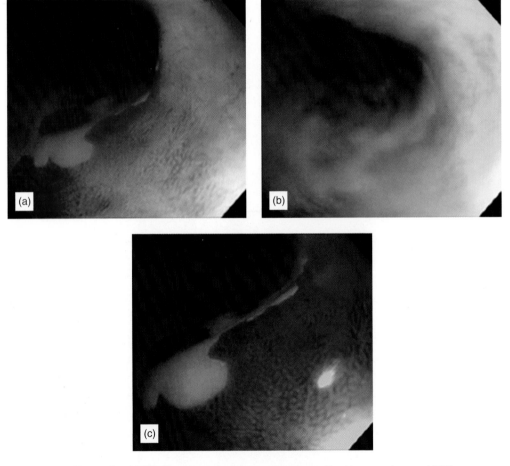

Figure 6.7 Example of NBI detection of a false positive autofluorescence image (AFI). (a) Unsuspicious area with high-resolution white light endoscopy. (b) AFI detects a purple appearing region, suspicious for dysplasia. In AFI, a purple colour indicates an area suspicious for neoplastic change in contrast to normal tissue which appears green. (c) Detailed inspection of this site with NBI reveals regular mucosal and vascular patterns that indicates that the AFI finding was a false positive. (with permission from Elsevier, Ref. [22]).

Section 2

Stomach and Duodenum

Clinical application of magnification endoscopy with NBI in the stomach and the duodenum

7

Kenshi Yao, Takashi Nagahama, Fumihito Hirai, Suketo Sou, Toshiyuki Matsui, Hiroshi Tanabe, Akinori Iwashita, Philip Kaye and Krish Ragunath

INTRODUCTION

Currently, within the stomach and the duodenum, there is no evidence to demonstrate the clinical usefulness of narrowband imaging (NBI) during non-magnifying endoscopic observation for the purpose of detecting abnormal pathology. However, several clinical applications are possible if NBI is applied to the magnification endoscopy technique in the stomach and the duodenum. Hence, in this chapter, we will describe the clinical usefulness of magnification endoscopy when used in conjuction with NBI.

BASIC PRINCIPLES FOR THE ANALYSIS OF MAGNIFIED ENDOSCOPIC FINDINGS

When analyzing the magnified endoscopic findings, there are two distinctly different anatomical findings which need to be examined [1]:
1 the subepithelial microvascular (MV) architecture;
2 the mucosal microsurface (MS) structure.
We should analyze these findings independently. By white light alone, only the MV architecture can be noted, but when we utilize NBI, both the MV architecture and the MS structure can be visualized.

MAGNIFICATION ENDOSCOPY PROCEDURE

The preparation of the patient for magnification endoscopy is the same as that for standard endoscopy. The endoscopy procedures described and illustrated in this article were performed using a high-resolution magnifying upper gastrointestinal (GI) endoscope (GIF-Q240Z, Olympus, Tokyo, Japan) and

Olympus-EVIS LUCERA SPECTRUM system. The structure-enhancement function of the video processor is set at a level of 4, 6 or 8 (level 4 or 6 for non-magnified observation and level 8 for magnified observation). Prior to endoscopy, a black soft hood (MB-162, Olympus, Tokyo) is attached to the tip of the scope (Figure 7.1) to enable the endoscopist to fix the focal distance at 3 mm between the tip of the scope and the mucosal surface at maximal magnification [2]. In practice, when a lesion on the gastric mucosa is found during non-magnifying observation, visualization of the lesion is immediately zoomed up to maximal magnification, and then the tip of the scope is allowed to contact the mucosa immediately after reaching the maximal magnification level. In this system, one can easily change the light source to either white light or NBI by using a button on the handle part of the scope.

THE STOMACH

In the stomach, the NBI technique is only useful when we apply this technique to magnification endoscopy. From a technical point of view, the mucosal image by non-magnification observation with NBI is too dark and noisy for meaningful investigation because the lumen of the stomach is large.

Normal gastric mucosa (Figs 7.2 and 7.3)

Basically, magnified endoscopic findings of normal gastric mucosa without any pathological change (such as *Helicobacter pylori* (HP) infection) are different depending upon the part of the stomach, that is, the gastric body or the gastric antrum [3–5].

With regard to the MV architecture in the normal gastric body (Figure 7.2a), it shows a honeycomb-like subepithelial capillary network (SECN) pattern with collecting venules (CV) (Figure 7.2b). More precisely, a polygonal loop of subepithelial capillary surrounds each gastric pit and these loops form a honeycomb-like network beneath the epithelium and converge onto a CV. By magnification with NBI, the MS structure becomes evident, namely, the pits demonstrate a round or oval shape (Figure 7.2c). If there is no pathological change such as HP gastritis in the mucosa, both the MV architecture and the MS structure constantly show a regular shape and arrangement [6–8].

On the other hand, the gastric antrum demonstrates distinctly different magnified endoscopic findings from those of the gastric body. In the MV architecture, the antral mucosa depicts a coil-shaped SECN (Figure 7.3b) [3]. CVs are rarely observed on the mucosal surface in the gastric antrum because anatomically the CV is thought to be located in a deeper part of the lamina propria in the gastric antrum than it is in the gastric body [5]. With regard to the MS structure of the gastric antrum, it also showed a quite different pattern from that of the gastric body. According to the classical convention, the gastric pits are thought to be round, but this idea is not correct. The pits demonstrate a linear or reticular pattern. Each coil-shaped subepithelial capillary is located in an apical part which is separated by a linear or reticular crypt-opening [3]. This characteristic MV architecture together with the MS structure can be clearly visualized when we apply NBI to magnification endoscopy (Figure 7.3c) (see DVD video clip 21).

Chronic gastritis

Magnification endoscopy has also been reported to be useful for identifying HP-associated gastritis and gastric atrophy (Figure 7.4) [6–8]. Briefly, the magnified endoscopic findings in the gastric body mucosa has been categorized into four types: type 1, honeycomb-like SECN with regular arrangement of CVs and regular round pits; type 2, honeycomb-like SECN with regular, round pits, but loss of CVs; type 3, loss of normal SECN and CVs, with enlarged white pits surrounded by erythema and type 4, loss of normal SECN and round pits together with an irregular arrangement of CVs [7]. Type 1 pattern is highly predictive for normal gastric mucosa with negative findings for HP infection. Type 2 or 3 pattern is predictive for an HP-infected stomach, while Type 4 pattern is predictive for gastric atrophy. This classification was made through modification of the original findings of both Yagi [6] and Nakagawa [8].

Uedo et al. reported an interesting concept and new application of NBI with magnifying endoscopy for the diagnosis of gastric intestinal metaplasia (Figure 7.5) [9]. They indicated that a distinctive finding called "light blue crest (LBC)" was a good indicator of histological intestinal metaplasia which is a risk factor for the development of differentiated (intestinal) type gastric cancer. The LBC was defined as a fine, blue-white line on the crests of the epithelial surface or gyri as visualized by magnification endoscopy with NBI. This appearance is speculated to be caused by reflection of the short and narrow wavelength light (400–430 nm) at the surface of the ciliated tissue structure, that is, the brush border in the gastric intestinal metaplasia and the duodenum. Current applications of this finding have not yet been established, however, it could play a key role in the approach to the pathogenesis of chronic metaplastic gastritis as visualized by endoscopy (see DVD video clip 22).

Differentiated carcinoma (intestinal type)
1. Disappearance of regular SECN pattern
2. A demarcation line (DL)
3. Irregular-micro vascular pattern (IMVP)
Undifferentiated carcinoma (diffuse type)
1. Reduced MV pattern

Table 7.1 Magnified endoscopic findings characteristic for early gastric cancer.

Early gastric cancer

Recently, we first reported unique magnified endoscopic findings based on MV architecture characteristics for early gastric cancer [2,3]. These findings were different depending upon the histological type, namely, differentiated carcinoma (intestinal type) or undifferentiated carcinoma (diffuse type) (Table 7.1).

With regard to differentiated carcinoma (Figure 7.6), briefly, the surrounding non-cancerous mucosa showed an SECN which was regular in both shape and arrangement. In contrast, the regular SECN pattern had disappeared at the margin of the carcinoma and instead microvessels which were irregular in both shape and arrangement had proliferated within the cancerous mucosa (irregular microvascular pattern, IMVP). In addition, a clear demarcation line (DL) could be noted between the cancerous and the non-cancerous mucosa. The presence of a DL and the disappearance of the regular SECN pattern were explained by the histological findings in which cancerous tissue replaces non-cancerous tissue when it extends horizontally.

Microvessels irregular in both shape and arrangement are thought to be tumorous vessels which have proliferated within the carcinomatous interstitial tissue, which shows irregularity in its histological findings. These findings were thought to be useful in clinical practice for making a correct diagnosis between superficial cancer and focal gastritis [10] and for determining the margin of the carcinoma prior to endoscopic resection [11,12]. On the other hand, with regard to undifferentiated carcinoma, the cancerous mucosa only showed reduced density of the SECN pattern (Figure 7.7). Other examples of how the information from HRE NBI with magnification can be used to differentiate between cancer and berign gastritis, as well as detect neoplasm which is invisible on standard endoscopy are shown in Figures 7.8–7.11. [see DVD video clips 23–26].

THE DUODENUM

Normal duodenal mucosa

By magnification endoscopy, finger- or leaf-like villi with a smooth surface which is regular in arrangement can be observed. NBI enables the endoscopist to obtain a clear view of the LBC at the edge of the villi and the intravillous capillary loop network (Figure 7.12) [see DVD video clip 32].

Celiac disease

Magnification endoscopy can enable the endoscopist not only to detect the villous atrophy [13], but also, to assess the degree of villous atrophy [14]. A scoring system (Z score) was proposed for grading the appearance of villous atrophy: "Z1" for normal mucosa, "Z2" for blunted villi, "Z3" for markedly blunted villi (with ridges and pits) and "Z4" for flat mucosa [14]. This scoring system seemed to be well correlated with histological assessment of villous atrophy. It was suggested that if we applied NBI to this magnification endoscopy, this grading system may remain accurate without the necessity for dye spraying, siince NBI can optically enhance both the MS structure and the MV architecture. Celiac disease is one of the promising indications for magnification endoscopy with NBI, as well illustrated by Figures 7.13–7.15.

CONCLUSION

Numerous findings by magnification endoscopy with NBI are still under investigation. Nevertheless, the most important advantage of this technique is that it can visualize both the MV architecture and the MS structure without the need to introduce any artificial materials (such as dye, etc.) into the human body. In the near future, magnification endoscopy with NBI is expected to be practiced as a standard endoscopy technique which is quick, safe and accurate for making a precise diagnosis of GI pathology.

ACKNOWLEDGEMENT

We wish to thank Miss Katherine Miller (Royal English Language Centre, Fukuoka, Japan) for revising the English.

REFERENCES

1. Yao K, Iwashita A. Clinical application of zoom endoscopy for the stomach (Japanese with English abstract). *Gastroenterol Endosc* 2006; 48: 1091–101.

2. Yao K, Oishi T, Matsui T, Yao T, Iwashita A. Novel magnified endoscopic findings of microvascular architecture in intramucosal gastric cancer. *Gastrointest Endosc* 2002; 56: 279–284.

3. Yao K, Oishi T. Microgastroscopic findings of mucosal microvascular architecture as visualized by magnifying endoscopy. *Dig Endosc* 2001; 13: S27–S33.

4. Yao K. Gastric microvascular architecture as visualized by magnifying endoscopy: body mucosa and antral mucosa without pathological change demonstrate two different patterns of microvascular architecture. *Gastrointest Endosc* 2004; 59: 596–597.

5. Gannon B. The vasculature and lymphatic drainage. In: Whitehead R, editor. *Gastrointestinal and Oesophageal Pathology*. Edinburgh: Churchill Livingstone, 1995, pp. 129–199.

6. Yagi K, Nakamura A, Sekine A. Characteristic endoscopic and magnified endoscopic findings in the normal stomach without *Helicobactor pylori* infection. *J Gastroenterol Hepatol* 2002; 17: 39–45.

7. Anagnostopoulos GK, Yao K, Kaye P, Fogden E, Fortun P, Shonde A, Foley S, Sunil S, Atherton J, Hawkey C, Ragunath K. High-resolution magnification endoscopy can reliably identify normal gastric mucosa, Helicobacter pylori-associated gastritis, and gastric atrophy. *Endoscopy* 2007; 39: 1–6.

8. Nakagawa S, Kato M, Shimizu Y, Nakagawa M, Yamamoto J, Luis PA, Kodaira J, Kawarasaki M, Takeda H, Sugiyama T, Asaka M. Relationship between histopathologic gastritis and mucosal microvascularity: observation with magnifying endoscopy. *Gastrointest Endosc* 2003; 58: 71–75.

9. Uedo N, Ishihara R, Iishi H, Yamamoto S, Yamamoto S, Yamada T, Imanaka K, Takeuchi Y, Higashino K, Ishiguro S, Tatsuta M. A new method of diagnosing gastric intestinal metaplasia: narrow band imaging with magnifying endoscopy. *Endoscopy* 2006; 38: 819–824.

10. Yao K, Iwashita A, Kikuchi Y, Yao T, Matsui T, Tanabe H, Nagahama T, Sou S, Hirai F. Novel zoom endoscopy technique for visualizing the microvascular architecture in gastric mucosa. *Clin Gastroenterol Hepatol* 2005; 3: S23–S26.

11. Yao K, Yao T, Iwashita A. Determining the horizontal extent of early gastric carcinoma: two modern techniques based on differences in the mucosal microvascular architecture and density between carcinoma and non-carcinomatous mucosa. *Dig Endosc* 2002; 14: S83–S87.

12. Yao K, Kikuchi Y, Tanabe H, Ikeda K, Iwashita A, Yorioka M, Sou S, Nagahama T, Wada Y, Yao T, Matsui T. Novel zoom-endoscopy technique for visualizing the microvascular architecture of early gastric cancer enables the precise margin of the cancer to be determined thereby allowing successful resection by the endoscopic submucosal dissection method. *Endoscopy* 2004; 36: A6.

13. Siegel LM, Stevens PD, Lightdale CJ, Green PH, Goodman S, Garcia-Carrasquillo RJ, Rotterdam H. Combined magnification endoscopy with chromoendoscopy in the evaluation of patients with suspected malabsorption. *Gastrointest Endosc* 1997; 46: 226–230.

14. Badreldin R, Barrett P, Wooff DA, Mansfield J, Yiannakou Y. How good is zoom endoscopy for assessment of villous atrophy in coeliac disease? *Endoscopy* 2005; 37: 994–998.

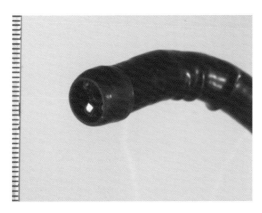

Figure 7.1 A black soft hood mounted at the tip of the scope (Copyright K. Yao, T. Nagahama, F. Hirai, S. Sou, T. Matsui, H. Tanbe, A. Iwashita, P. Kaye, K. Ragunath).

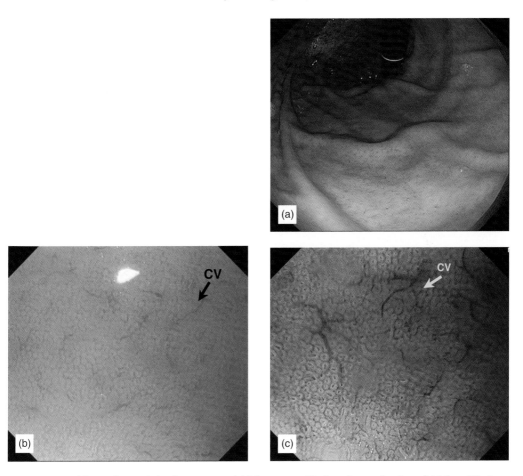

Figure 7.2 Normal gastric body mucosa. (a) Non-magnified endoscopic view. (b) Magnified endoscopic findings by white light. A honeycomb-like SECN pattern with CV, arrow can be noted. (c) Magnified endoscopic findings by NBI. In addition to the microvasculature, a round or oval pit pattern becomes evident. The MV architecture and MS structure appear regular in both shape and arrangement in the normal gastric body mucosa (Copyright K. Yao, T. Nagahama, F. Hirai, S. Sou, T. Matsui, H. Tanbe, A. Iwashita, P. Kaye, K. Ragunath).

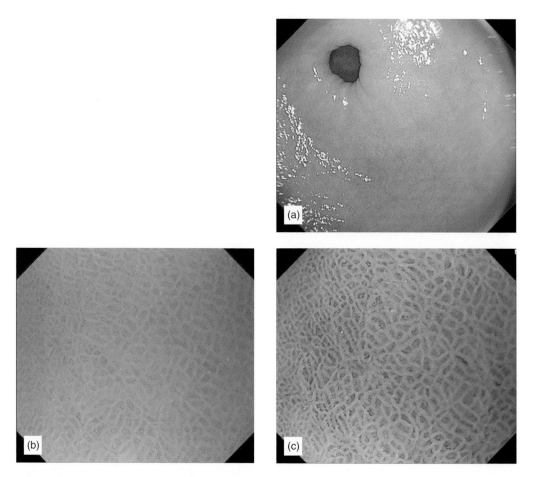

Figure 7.3 Normal gastric antral mucosa. (a) Non-magnified endoscopic view. (b) Magnified endoscopic findings by white light. A coil-shaped SECN pattern is present. (c) Magnified endoscopic findings by NBI. Both the coil-shaped SECN pattern and the reticular MS structure are clearly demonstrated by NBI (Copyright K. Yao, T. Nagahama, F. Hirai, S. Sou, T. Matsui, H. Tanabe, A. Iwashita, P. Kaye, K. Ragunath).

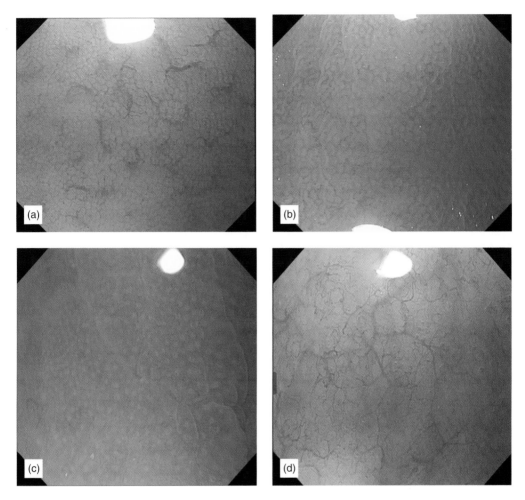

Figure 7.4 Magnified endoscopic views of the gastric mucosa according to the classification of HP-associated gastritis. (a) Type 1, honeycomb-like SECN with regular arrangement of CVs and regular round pits. (b) Type 2, honeycomb-like SECN with regular, round pits, but loss of CVs. (c) Type 3, loss of normal SECN and CVs, with enlarged white pits surrounded by erythema. (d) Type 4, loss of normal SECN and round pits, and together with an irregular arrangement of CVs (Copyright K. Yao, T. Nagahama, F. Hirai, S. Sou, T. Matsui, H. Tanabe, A. Iwashita, P. Kaye, K. Ragunath).

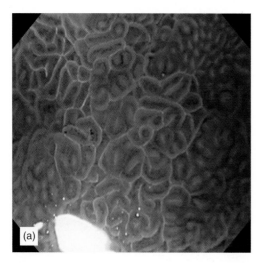

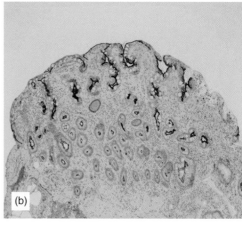

Figure 7.5 (a) Magnified endoscopic findings of "Light blue crests" (LBC) in the gastric antral mucosa. LBC is clearly visualized as blue-white lines on the epithelial edge or surface by magnification with NBI. (b) Histological findings of a biopsy specimen from the area that is positive for LBC (immunostain, CD10). The epithelial surface with intestinal metaplasia and goblet cells is strongly stained by CD10. (The images of Figure 7.5a and 7.5b were kindly provided by Dr. N. Uedo, Osaka Medical Center for Cancer and Cardiovascular Diseases, Osaka, Japan.) (Copyright K. Yao, T. Nagahama, F. Hirai, S. Sou, T. Matsui, H. Tanabe, A. Iwashita, P. Kaye, K. Ragunath).

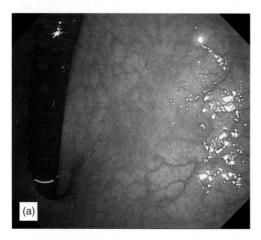

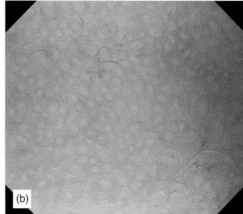

Figure 7.6 An example of an early gastric cancer in the gastric cardia. (a) On ordinary white light endoscopy, a flat reddened mucosal lesion can be noted. (b) Magnification endoscopy with white light shows a regular SECN pattern of the non-cancerous surrounding mucosa.

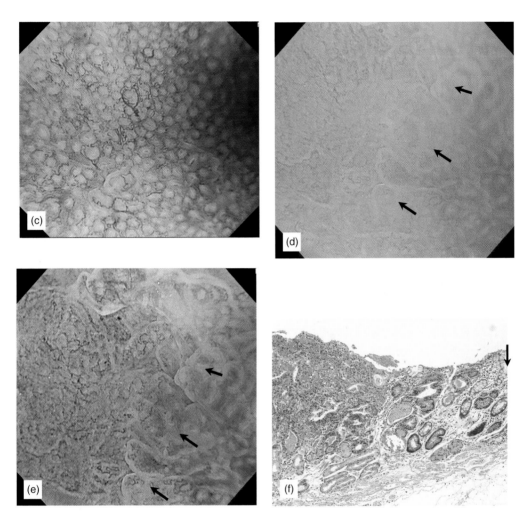

Figure 7.6 (Continued) (c) With NBI, the regular shape and arrangement of the capillaries together with the pit pattern become evident. (d) At the margin of the carcinoma, white light magnification endoscopy shows a DL (arrows). At that location, the regular SECN pattern has disappeared and, instead, microvessels which are irregular in both shape and arrangement can be seen to have proliferated within the cancerous mucosa. (e) When the white light imaging is changed to NBI, the characteristic findings for differentiated carcinoma (such as the presence of a DL (arrows) and an irregular microvascular pattern (IMVP) become distinct. (f) Histological findings (Hematoxylin & Eosin, HE stain) of the endoscopically resected specimen demonstrate well-differentiated adenocarcinoma replacing the non-cancerous tissue. An arrow shows the histological margin between cancerous and non-cancerous tissues (Copyright K. Yao, T. Nagahama, F. Hirai, S. Sou, T. Matsui, H. Tanabe, A. Iwashita, P. Kaye, K. Ragunath).

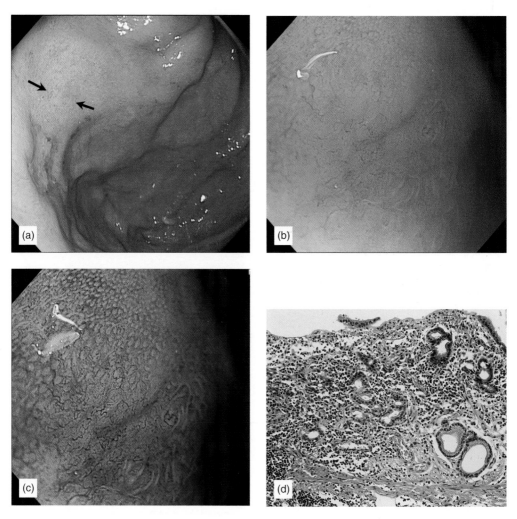

Figure 7.7 An example of early gastric cancer of undifferentiated type in the gastric fundus. (a) Ordinary white light endoscopic view shows a pale mucosal area (arrows) with ulceration. (b) Magnification endoscopic findings of that pale mucosa only show loss of the regular SECN pattern. (c) With NBI, flat mucosa with loss of the regular SECN is easily visualized. (d) Histopathological findings (HE stain) demonstrate that poorly differentiated adenocarci–nomatous cells are infiltrating within the lamina propria without any proliferation of interstitial tissue and that they are destroying the non-cancerous interstitial tissues (Copyright K. Yao, T. Nagahama, F. Hirai, S. Sou, T. Matsui, H. Tanabe, A. Iwashita, P. Kaye, K. Ragunath).

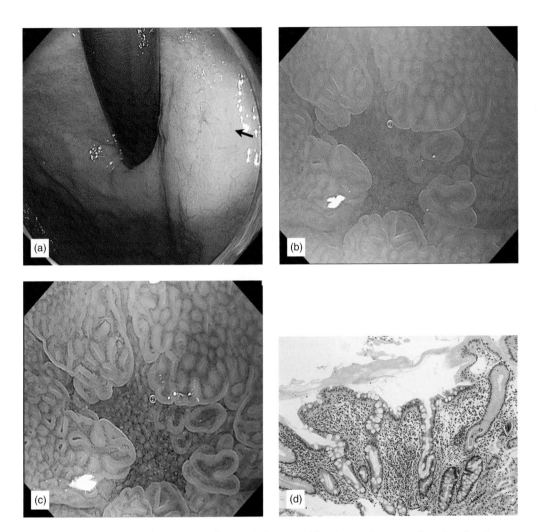

Figure 7.8 How to make a correct diagnosis by magnification endoscopy: Case 1, a focal mucosal lesion due to gastritis. (a) A slightly reddened depressed lesion with an irregularly shaped margin can be noted within the upper part of the gastric body. (b) When we observe this lesion at maximal magnification with white light, some of the MV network within the depressed part becomes visible. However, it is difficult to determine whether or not the shape and the arrangement of the microvessels are regular by these findings alone. (c) When we switch from white light to NBI, both the MV network and the pit pattern prove to be regular in both shape and arrangement. Accordingly, these findings are compatible with chronic focal gastritis. (d) The histopathological findings demonstrate only chronic gastritis with intestinal metaplasia (Copyright K. Yao, T. Nagahama, F. Hirai, S. Sou, T. Matsui, H. Tanabe, A. Iwashita, P. Kaye, K. Ragunath).

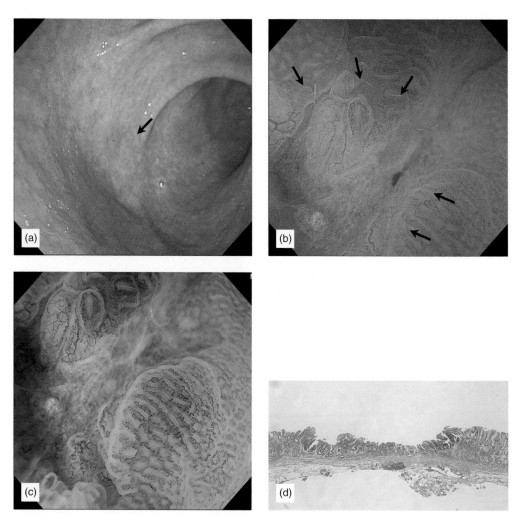

Figure 7.9 How to make a correct diagnosis by magnification endoscopy: Case 2, a small gastric cancer. (a) A slightly reddened depressed lesion with an irregularly shaped margin can be detected within the gastric antrum. (b) When we magnify this lesion, an IMVP can be identified within the depressed part (arrows). (c) With NBI, the distinct morphology of each of the micro-vessels can be observed in higher contrast than with white light. In addition, the mucosal surface of the depressed part depicts unevenness. (d) Histopathological findings of the endoscopically resected specimen represent a well-differentiated adenocarcinoma restricted to the mucosa (Copyright K. Yao, T. Nagahama, F. Hirai, S. Sou, T. Matsui, H. Tanabe, A. Iwashita, P. Kaye, K. Ragunath).

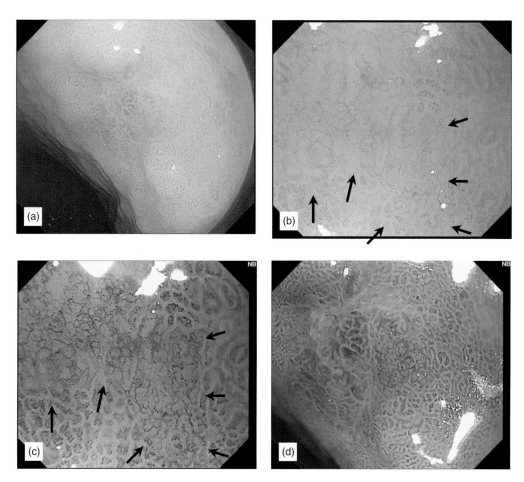

Figure 7.10 How to determine the precise margins of the carcinoma for successful resection by the endoscopic submucosal dissection (ESD) method. (a) A small, poorly demarcated mucosal lesion can be noted in the gastric body. (b) By magnification with white light, there is a DL; furthermore, at that part, the regular SECN pattern has disappeared and instead microvessels which are irregular in both shape and arrangement can be seen to have proliferated. (c) With NBI, these magnified endoscopic findings characteristic for differentiated carcinoma become easy to identify.

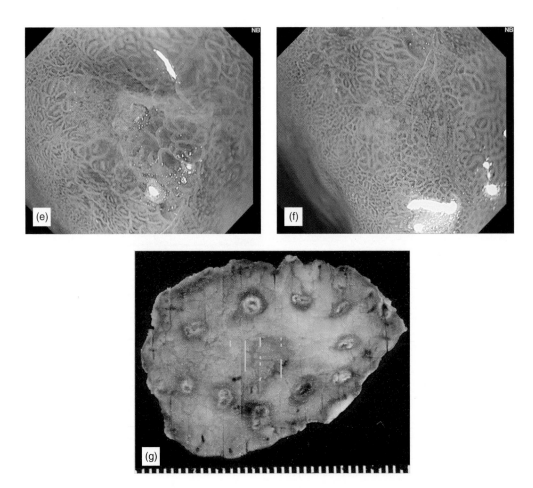

Figure 7.10 (Continued) (d–f) Once these magnified endoscopic findings characteristic for carcinoma are verified, all the margins of the carcinoma can be determined even at weak magnification, by endoscopic findings alone. (g) According to the histological investigation, the area of the carcinoma was reconstructed on the specimen which was resected by the ESD method. We can see that the reconstructed area is well correlated to that determined by magnification endoscopy with NBI (Copyright K. Yao, T. Nagahama, F. Hirai, S. Sou, T. Matsui, H. Tanabe, A. Iwashita, P. Kaye, K. Ragunath).

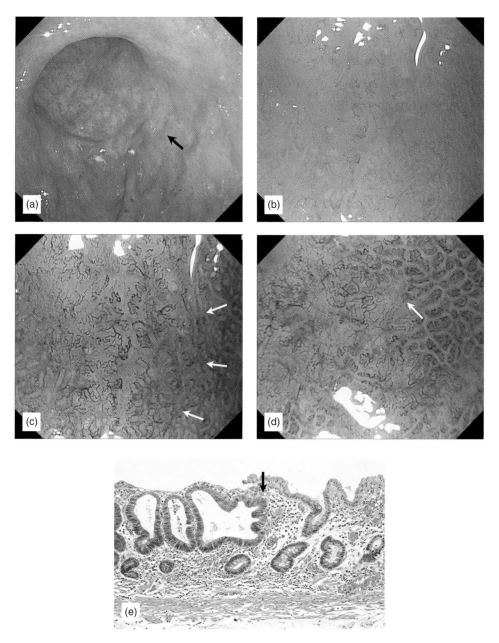

Figure 7.11 How to identify the presence of a carcinoma which does not show any macroscopic findings by ordinary endoscopy (so-called "occult cancer"). (a) One of the multiple random biopsies which were previously taken from the lower gastric body mucosa of the greater curvature was known to have represented well-differentiated adenocarcinoma. However, ordinary endoscopic findings only show multiple healed ulcers on the rough mucosa in the lower gastric body. (b) Instead of taking a second round of multiple biopsies, we scanned this area by weak magnification and successfully found the presence of the carcinoma by identifying an IMVP. (c, d) With NBI, the contrast of microvessels became remarkably high. Such high-contrast images enable the endoscopist to clearly identify a DL (arrows) between the non-cancerous and the cancerous mucosa, as well as an IMVP within the cancerous mucosa. These techniques may be useful in helping endoscopists avoid the need to take additional multiple biopsies. (e) Histopathological findings of the specimen which was resected by the ESD method demonstrate well-differentiated adenocarcinoma which was limited to the mucosa. An arrow shows the margin of the carcinoma (Copyright K. Yao, T. Nagahama, F. Hirai, S. Sou, T. Matsui, H. Tanabe, A. Iwashita, P. Kaye, K. Ragunath).

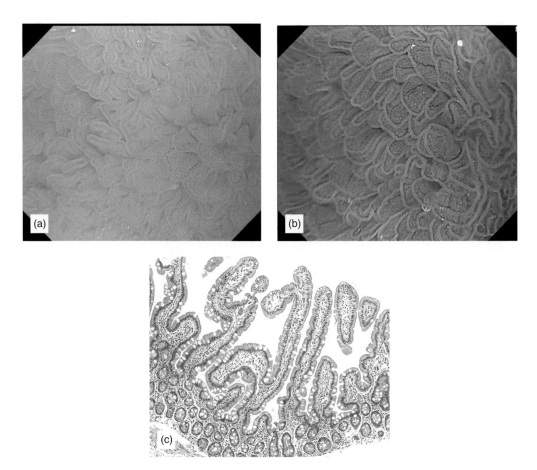

Figure 7.12 The normal duodenal mucosa. (a) Magnified endoscopic findings with white light. The finger- or leaf-like villous formation with a smooth edge is arranged in a regular manner. (b) By NBI, the MS structure of the villi and the MV architecture within the villi become distinct. At the edge of the villi, the Light blue crests (LBC) are visualized by NBI. Together, the capillary loops form a regular network underneath the epithelium within the villi (intravillous capillary loop network). (c) Histological findings of the biopsy specimen show no villous atrophy and no significant inflammatory infiltrate (Copyright K. Yao, T. Nagahama, F. Hirai, S. Sou, T. Matsui, H. Tanabe, A. Iwashita, P. Kaye, K. Ragunath).

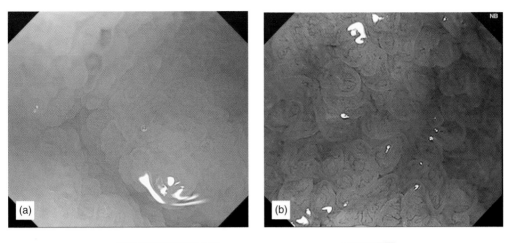

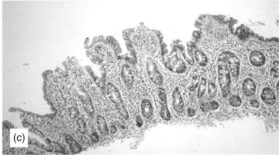

Figure 7.13 Duodenal mucosa in a patient with celiac disease. (a) Magnified endoscopic findings with white light. Blunted villi can be noted. (b) By NBI, the precise morphology of the villi can been seen; that is, the villi are blunted but the villous structure is still preserved. (c) Histological findings of the biopsy specimen demonstrate duodenal mucosa with mild partial villous atrophy (Copyright K. Yao, T. Nagahama, F. Hirai, S. Sou, T. Matsui, H. Tanabe, A. Iwashita, P. Kaye, K. Ragunath).

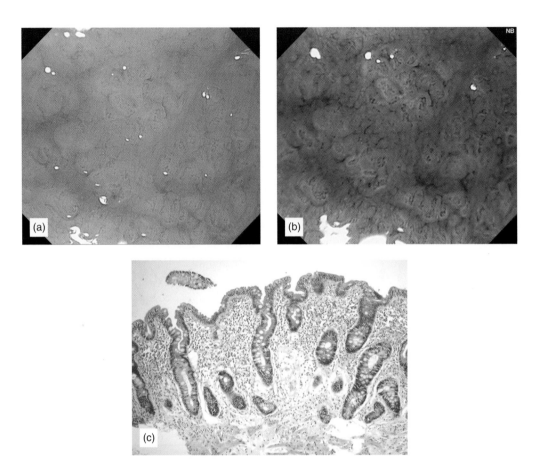

Figure 7.14 Duodenal mucosa in a patient with celiac disease. (a) Magnified endoscopic findings with white light demonstrate that the normal finger- or leaf-like villi have disappeared, but remarkably blunted villi are present. (b) NBI is helpful for visualizing the detailed MS structure, that is, blunted and broad villi with ridges and crypt-openings. (c) The histological findings of the biopsy specimen represent subtotal villous atrophy and chronic inflammatory infiltration into the epithelium and the lamina propria mucosa (Copyright K. Yao, T. Nagahama, F. Hirai, S. Sou, T. Matsui, H. Tanabe, A. Iwashita, P. Kaye, K. Ragunath).

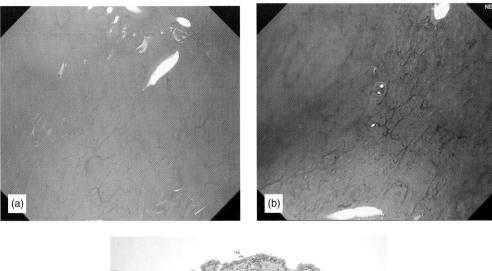

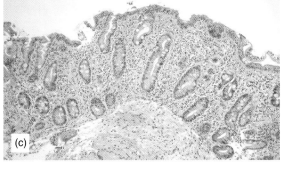

Figure 7.15 The duodenal mucosa in a patient with celiac disease. (a) Magnified endoscopic findings with white light show flat mucosa where the normal villous structure together with the normal microvasculature has disappeared. (b) In addition, NBI is useful for detecting even a small tubular crypt-openings on the surface of the flat mucosa. (c) By histological investigation of the biopsy specimen, it is evident that almost all of the villi have disappeared, and only a tubular appearance can be noted. Remarkable infiltration of chronic inflammatory cells into the lamina propria and the epithelium is also present (Copyright K. Yao, T. Nagahama, F. Hirai, S. Sou, T. Matsui, H. Tanabe, A. Iwashita, P. Kaye, K. Ragunath).

8

Magnifying endoscopy with NBI in the diagnosis of superficial gastric neoplasia and its application for ESD

Mitsuru Kaise, Takashi Nakayoshi and Hisao Tajiri

THE HISTORY OF MAGNIFYING ENDOSCOPY AND THE IMPACT OF NARROWBAND IMAGING ON MAGNIFYING ENDOSCOPIC DIAGNOSIS FOR GASTRIC NEOPLASIA

Although magnifying endoscopic diagnosis for gastric neoplasia has been attempted in the past decades [1], standardized systemic classification of magnified gastric surface has not been established due to diverse histology of gastric carcinomas, the existence of three different types of proper gastric mucosa (Figure 8.1), and various modifications on mucosal structures by atrophy, chronic inflammation and metaplasia (Figure 8.2). The development of magnifying video-endoscopy combined with narrowband imaging (NBI) has broken this situation and opened a new door. NBI yields very clear images of fine superficial structure as well as microvasculature of the gastric mucosa (Figure 8.3), which has advanced magnifying endoscopic diagnosis into a new stage. We have reported that significant correlation between histopathology and microvascular pattern obtained with NBI enables the sensitive diagnosis for the existence [2] and extent of superficial gastric cancer, and therefore the modality is applicable for endoscopic submucosal dissection (ESD) [3].

FINDINGS OF MICROVASCULATURE ON DIAGNOSIS OF SUPERFICIAL DEPRESSED GASTRIC CANCER

We have done a prospective study to measure the correlation between the magnified images obtained with NBI and the histological findings, especially with regard to the microvascular pattern; 225 cases of superficial depressed gastric carcinoma (152 of well-differentiated adenocarcinoma and 75 of poorly differentiated adenocarcinomas) were enrolled in the study.

The mixed type with well and poorly differentiated adenocarcinoma recognized in 27 cases was classified into one of the types according to the prominant histological characteristic. Microvascular patterns on the mucosal surface were classified into two patterns: fine network pattern and corkscrew pattern (Figure 8.4). The fine network pattern appears as a mesh, and abundant microvessels are well connected with one another. In contrast, the corkscrew pattern has isolated and tortuous microvessels, and accordingly appears like a corkscrew. The mixed type with both network and corkscrew patterns was classified into one of the types according to the prominant finding.

Fine network pattern was recognized in 104 cases (68.4%) of 152 well-differentiated adenocarcinomas (intestinal type). Corkscrew pattern was observed in 64 cases (85.3%) of 75 poorly differentiated adenocarcinoma (diffuse type) (Table 8.1). In 50 lesions, microvascular findings were not obtained due to viscid mucus, bleeding or an unclassified type of microvessel. The evidence indicates that the presence and histology of superficial gastric carcinoma can be predicated by the microvascular patterns, suggesting that the magnified videoendoscopy with NBI system could achieve optical biopsy.

We also used a standard microscope and a laser scanning microscope (LSM) to observe gastric cancerous mucosa by CD31 specific to the vascular endothelium cell, in order to compare the three-dimensional construction of microvessels with histological characteristics. In well-differentiated adenocarcinoma, networks of microvessels run around cancerous glands since the glandular structures were kept in shape (Figure 8.5). In contrast, in poorly differentiated adenocarcinoma, isolated corkscrew-like microvessels randomly and chaotically exist due to the lack of glandular structure that normally restricts the space for vessels to run (Figure 8.6). Microvessel images obtained by LSM, and the ones by magnifying endoscopy with NBI had a good correlation (Figures 8.5 and 8.6). Therefore, microvessel images obtained by magnifying endoscopy with NBI may correspond well to the histological characteristics which ensures the possibility of optical biopsy.

	Fine net pattern	Corkscrew pattern	Unclassified type/no findings
Well-differentiated carcinoma (152 cases)	104 cases (68.4%)	7 cases (4.6%)	41 cases (27.0%)
Poorly differentiated carcinoma (75 cases)	2 cases (2.7%)	64 cases (85.3%)	9 cases (12.0%)

Table 8.1 Comparison of microvascular patterns and histological characteristics in superficial depressed gastric carcinoma.

For the magnifying endoscopic diagnosis of superficial depressed gastric carcinoma, both the existence of irregular microvessels and the disappearance of fine superficial structure are essential. A cancerous depression with irregular microvessels and structural disappearance can be distinctly differentiated from non-neoplastic mucosa with fine superficial structure by a definite borderline. The borderline is almost comparable to the demarcation line proposed by Yao [4], which was reported to be observable in depressed gastric cancers composed of well-differentiated adenocarcinoma, but not in those of poorly differentiated adenocarcinoma. However, we consider that the borderline between cancerous depression and non-neoplastic surrounding mucosa is observable both in well and poorly differentiated adenocarcinoma, if you take account of the differences both in microvessel and fine superficial structure.

FINDINGS OF MAGNIFYING ENDOSCOPY IN SUPERFICIAL ELEVATED NEOPLASIAS OF THE STOMACH

The microvascular classification established in superficial depressed neoplasias cannot be simply applied to superficial elevated neoplasias due to the lack of visibility of microvessels. Therefore, in elevated gastric lesions, magnifying endoscopic diagnosis is based on microvessels as well as fine mucosal structures. In gastric adenoma, fine mucosal patterns are able to be classified to tubular, round or oval shapes, and irregularity is rarely recognized in the microvascular and fine mucosal patterns (Figure 8.11). On the other hand, irregularity in fine mucosal pattern and microvessel can be observed in superficial elevated gastric carcinoma (type 0 IIa), and therefore findings with NBI are useful in diagnosing gastric elevated lesions; however, irregular microvessels are not frequently recognized in elevated carcinomas [5]. In cases without irregular mucosal structure and microvessel, indigo carmine dye is often useful to identify the extent of cancer. Thus it is better to use both methods for ESD/endoscopic mucosal resection (EMR) marking (Figures 8.7–8.13).

APPLICATION OF MAGNIFYING ENDOSCOPY WITH NBI ON ENDOSCOPIC RESECTION

The diagnosis of the extent of cancerous infiltration is indispensable for endoscopic or surgical resection of gastric carcinoma. Since around 20% of superficial gastric carcinomas do not give a clear borderline, accurate endoscopic diagnosis plays a crucial role for a radical cure, especially in endoscopic resection. ESD, a recently developed superb method which enables an en bloc resection for large lesions, can achieve more radical cure in combination with precise endoscopic diagnosis of the cancerous extent. Therefore, we usually perform ESD in combination with magnifying endoscopy with NBI, which can allow real time optical biopsy [2] [see DVD video clips 28 and 29].

REFERENCES

1. Sakaki N, Iida Y, Okazaki Y, Kawamura S, Takemoto T. Magnifying endoscopic observation of the gastric mucosa, particularly in patients with atrophic gastritis. *Endoscopy* 1978; 10: 269–274.
2. Nakayoshi T, Tajiri H, Matsuda K, Kaise M, Ikegami M, Sasaki H. Magnifying endoscopy combined with narrow band imaging system for early gastric cancer: correlation of vascular pattern with histopathology (including video). *Endoscopy* 2004; 36: 1080–1084.
3. Sumiyama K, Kaise M, Nakayoshi T, Kato M, Mashiko T, Uchiyama Y, et al. Combined use of a magnifying endoscope with a narrow band imaging system and a multibending endoscope for en bloc EMR of early stage gastric cancer. *Gastrointest Endosc* 2004; 60: 79–84.
4. Yao K, Oishi T, Matsui T, Yao T, Iwashita A. Novel magnified endoscopic findings of microvascular architecture in intramucosal gastric cancer. *Gastrointest Endosc* 2002; 56: 279–284.
5. Nakayoshi T, Tajiri H, Saitoh S, Matsuda K, Mochizuki K, Kaise M, et al. Magnifying endoscopic diagnosis of gastric adenoma (Japanese). *I to Chyo* 2003; 38: 1401–1409.

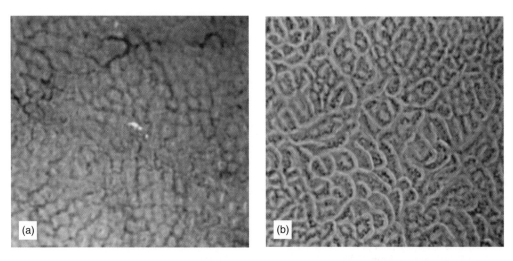

Figure 8.1 Normal mucosal images obtained by magnifying endoscopy with NBI. (a) Mucosal surface of gastric fundic gland; there appear microvessels surrounding the gland pits, which shows a honeycomb pattern. (b) Mucosal surface of pyloric gland; there appear microvessels surrounding the tubular type pit and stripe pit. Microvessels observed in cancerous lesions have irregularity; abnormal dilatation, abrupt alteration in caliber and heterogeneity in shape. In contrast, microvessels observed in non-neoplastic mucosa surround along mucosal pits and have regularity; similarity in shape and even alteration in caliber (Copyright M. Kaise, T. Nakayoshi, H. Tajiri).

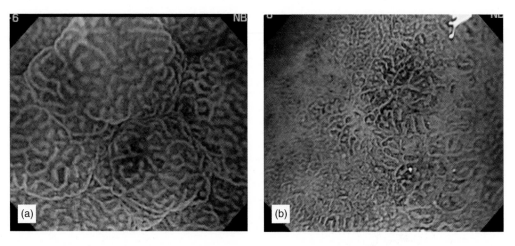

Figure 8.2 Modifications on mucosal structures by atrophy, chronic inflammation and meta-plasia. (a) *Helicobacter pylori*-infected fundic mucosa demonstrates round, tubular or gyrus-like patterns of fine superficial structure, which is different from normal fundic mucosa with regular round pit pattern and honeycomb-like microvessels (Figure 8.1(a)). (b) In *Helicobacter pylori*-infected pyloric mucosa, patterns of fine superficial structures are various, and invisible in atrophic mucosa. Microvessels surround the various shapes of superficial structure, and the density of microvessels varies from area to area (Copyright M. Kaise, T. Nakayoshi, H. Tajiri).

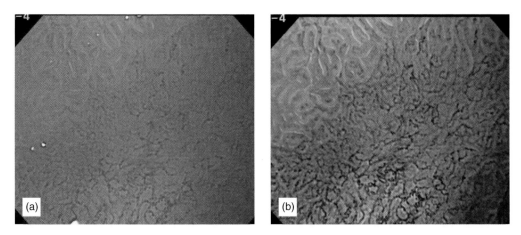

Figure 8.3 Comparison of (a) white light magnifying endoscopy and (b) magnifying endoscopy with NBI (Copyright M. Kaise, T. Nakayoshi, H. Tajiri).

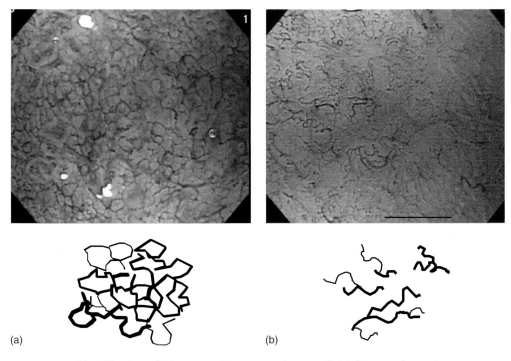

Figure 8.4 Classification of microvascular patterns in superficial depressed gastric cancer. (a) Fine network pattern looks like a mesh, in which abundant microvessels connect with one another. (b) Corkscrew pattern has isolated and tortuous microvessels, in which scanty microvessels do not connect with one another. The vessels in cancerous lesions show abnormal dilatation, abrupt alteration in caliber and heterogeneity in shape. Fine mucosal structures usually disappear in depressed gastric carcinoma (Copyright M. Kaise, T. Nakayoshi, H. Tajiri).

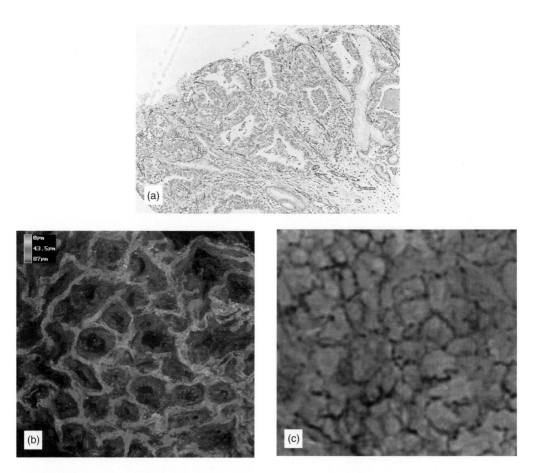

Figure 8.5 Images of microvessels in well-differentiated (intestinal type) adenocarcinoma. (a) CD31-immunostainined, optical microscope findings: microvessels surrounding cancerous glands. (b) CD31-immunostaining: the three-dimensional structures of the microvessels displayed by LSM show the presence of network of microvessels. (c) There is a good correlation between microvascular patterns demonstrated by magnifying endoscopy with NBI and those by LSM (Copyright M. Kaise, T. Nakayoshi, H. Tajiri).

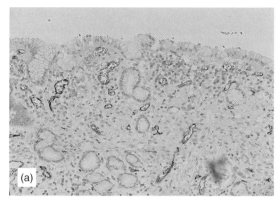

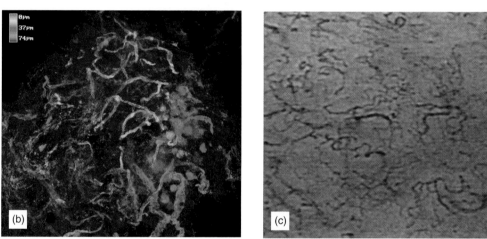

Figure 8.6 Images of microvessels in poorly differentiated (diffuse type) adenocarcinoma. (a) CD31-immunostainined, optical microscope findings: microvessels are present. They are isolated and randomly arranged due to the lack of glandular structure which restricts vessels to run freely. (b) CD31-immunostainined: the three-dimensional structures of the microvessels displayed by LSM show the presence of corkscrew network. (c) There is a good correlation between microvascular patterns displayed by magnifying endoscopy with NBI and the those by LSM (Copyright M. Kaise, T. Nakayoshi, H. Tajiri).

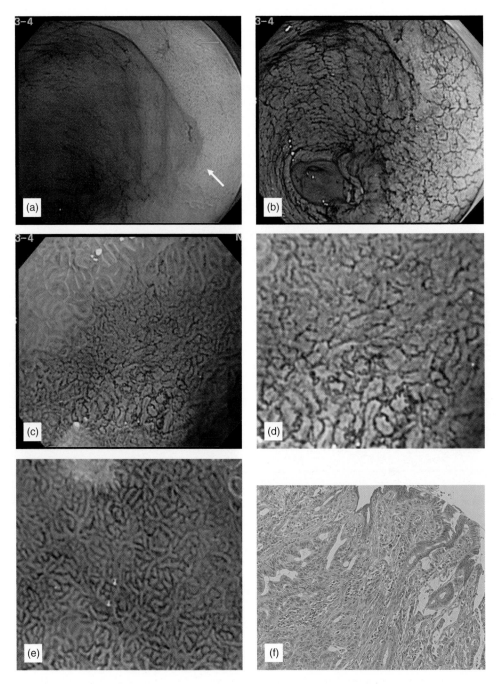

Figure 8.7 Type 0 IIc early gastric cancer of well-differentiated adenocarcinoma. The conventional endoscopy (a) and the chromoendoscopy (b) show the presence of two reddish and erosive lesions on the posterior wall of gastric antrum. It is still difficult to recognize the gastric erosions as cancerous or not. Magnifying endoscopy with NBI demonstrates the depressed lesion (white arrow in (a)) to have no fine mucosal patterns, but fine network microvessels, indicating that it is a well-differentiated adenocarcinoma ((c): medium magnification, (d): high magnification). (e) Magnifying endoscopy with NBI demonstrates the other depressed lesion (blue arrow in (a)) to have tubular mucosal pattern and regular microvessels, indicating that the lesion is non-cancerous erosion. (f) Pathological findings of the early gastric cancer shows well-differentiated adenocarcinoma (intestinal type), which is in accordance with the histology prediction by magnifying endoscopy with NBI (Copyright M. Kaise, T. Nakayoshi, H. Tajiri).

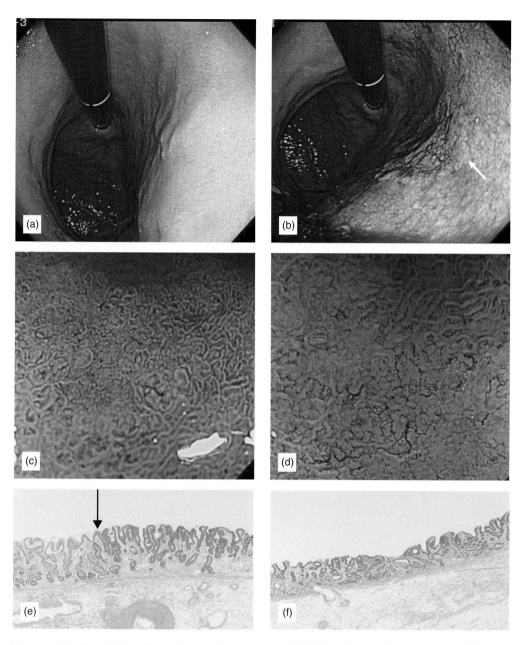

Figure 8.8 Type 0 IIc + IIa early gastric cancer of well-differentiated adenocarcinoma. The conventional endoscopy shows discolored lesions (a) on the anterior wall of upper gastric corpus and the chromoendoscopy (b) clearly shows the 3 cm superficial depressed lesions with surrounding elevation, indicating the possibility of the early gastric cancer. (c) Magnifying endoscopy with NBI (medium magnification) shows a slightly depressed area with very small mucosal pattern. (d) High magnification shows a fine network of microvessels with abnormal dilatation, abrupt alteration in caliber and heterogeneity in shape. These findings indicate that the lesion is superficial well-differentiated adenocarcinoma. Pathological image of ESD specimen (e) shows type 0 IIa with a marginal edge to the right side of the black arrow and the left side shows a non-cancerous area. (f) shows pathological image of type 0 IIc in the center of the lesion, which is well-differentiated adenocarcinoma in accordance with the histological prediction by magnifying endoscopy with NBI (Copyright M. Kaise, H. Tajiri).

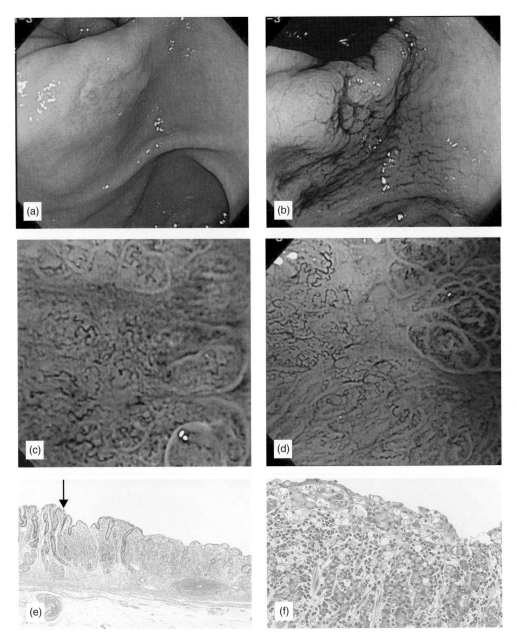

Figure 8.9 Type 0 IIc early gastric cancer of poorly differentiated adenocarcinoma. The conventional endoscopy shows discolored depressed lesions with reddish granulation on the posterior wall of gastric angle (a), and the chromoendoscopy with indigo carmine dye (b) shows the clearer appearance, of which morphology suggests the possibility of poorly differentiated adenocarcinoma. Magnifying endoscopy with NBI shows no mucosal pattern but irregular microvessels with corkscrew pattern, indicating that it is a well-differentiated adenocarcinoma. (c) Medium magnification. (d) High magnification. Upper right part of (d) is equal to the slightly elevated part with granulation which exists in the center of the lesion. This finding suggests that the area is not comprised of cancerous tissue in all the layers, but is covered with regenerated epithelium. Pathological findings of ESD specimen. (e) Magnifying endoscopy shows type 0 IIc to the right side of the black arrow. (f) High-magnified image of Hematoxylin and Eosin (H&E) histopathology shows poorly differentiated adenocarcinoma, which is in accordance with the histological prediction by magnifying endoscopy with NBI (Copyright M. Kaise, T. Nakayoshi, H. Tajiri).

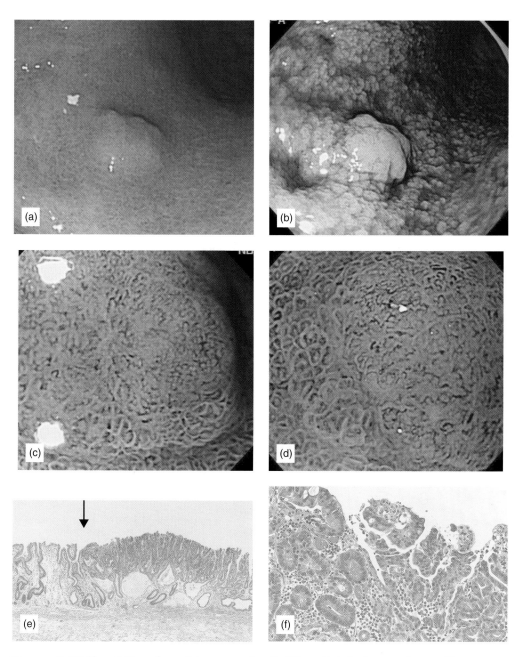

Figure 8.10 Type 0 IIa early gastric cancer of well-differentiated adenocarcinoma. The conventional endoscopy (a) and the chromoendoscopy (b) show a superficial elevated lesion with redness in the center. It is still difficult to judge whether the lesion is gastric adenoma or gastric cancer. Magnifying endoscopy with NBI (c) shows small-round mucosal pattern and microvessels with little heterogeneity in shape and no abrupt alteration in caliber. However (d) shows irregular microvessels with heterogeneous shape and uneven caliber, providing the diagnosis of type 0 IIa of well-differentiated adenocarcinoma. Pathological findings of ESD specimens. (e) shows type 0 IIa early gastric cancer to the right side of the black arrow. (f) High-magnified image shows well-differentiated adenocarcinoma, which is in accordance with the histological prediction by magnifying endoscopy with NBI (Copyright M. Kaise, T. Nakayoshi, H. Tajiri).

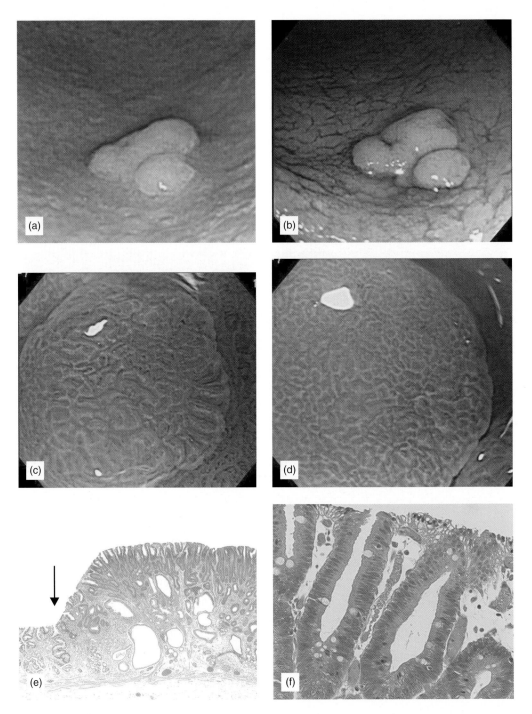

Figure 8.11 Gastric adenoma. The conventional endoscopy (a) and the chromoendoscopy (b), show a superficial elevated lesion composed of a few nodules on the gastric angle, which suggests the lesion to be a gastric adenoma. Magnifying endoscopy with NBI shows regular tubular mucosal patterns (c) and small-round mucosal patterns (d), but no irregular microvessels, suggesting the diagnosis of gastric adenoma. Pathologic findings of ESD specimen: (e) shows slightly elevated tumorous lesion to the right side of the black arrow, and (f) high-magnified image shows tubular adenoma with moderate atypia, which is in accordance with the histological prediction by magnifying endoscopy with NBI (Copyright M. Kaise, T. Nakayoshi, H. Tajiri).

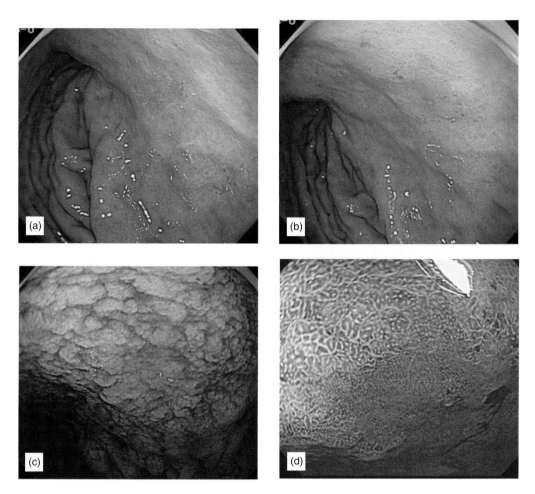

Figure 8.12 Type 0 IIc early gastric cancer of which existence or extent diagnosis of neoplastic infiltration is difficult. The conventional endoscopy only shows a reddish area on the posterior wall of upper gastric corpus with thickened mucus (a). Washing the mucus off provides the image of superficial depressed lesion in a reddish mucosa but still it is difficult to diagnose as gastric cancer (b). The chromoendoscopy with indigo carmine dye (c) suggests structural differences between the slightly depressed area and the surrounding mucosa, but still could not give the qualitative diagnosis of cancer. Magnifying endoscopy with NBI (d) shows that its mucosal pattern is smaller than the surrounding mucosa, and the depressed area has abundant microvessels.

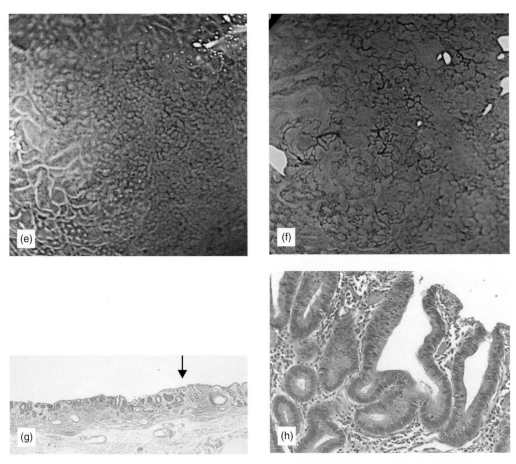

Figure 8.12 (Continued) The medium-magnified image (e) shows microvessels with network pattern on the depressed area. The high-magnified image (f) shows the irregular microvessels with fine network pattern, which could provide the diagnosis of type 0 IIc early gastric cancer of well-differentiated adenocarcinoma. Pathological findings of ESD specimen: (g) shows a neoplastic lesion to the left side of the black arrow, which is even in mucosal height as compared to surrounding non-neoplastic mucosa, meaning the lesion is type 0 IIb early gastric cancer. (h) High-magnified image shows well-differentiated adenocarcinoma, which is in accordance with the histological prediction by magnifying endoscopy with NBI (Copyright M. Kaise, T. Nakayoshi, H. Tajiri).

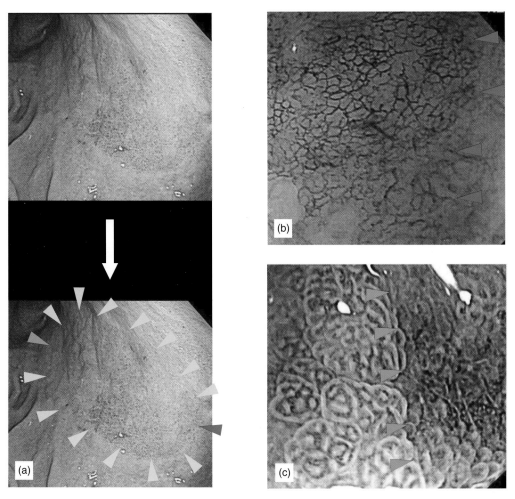

Figure 8.13 Gastric cancer of which existence or extent diagnosis is difficult by conventional endoscopy. (a) Conventional endoscopy shows a reddish area on the posterior wall of the upper gastric corpus but it is still difficult to diagnosis as a cancerous lesion. By magnifying endoscopy with NBI, it could be diagnosed as an early gastric cancer pointed out by arrowheads (type 0 IIc + IIb, well-differentiated adenocarcinoma). (b) Magnifying endoscopy with NBI shows irregular microvessels with the margin pointed out by the green arrowheads, indicating that the lesion is well-differentiated adenocarcinoma. (c) Magnifying endoscopy with NBI shows a slight depression and irregular microvessels with the margin pointed out by blue arrowheads.

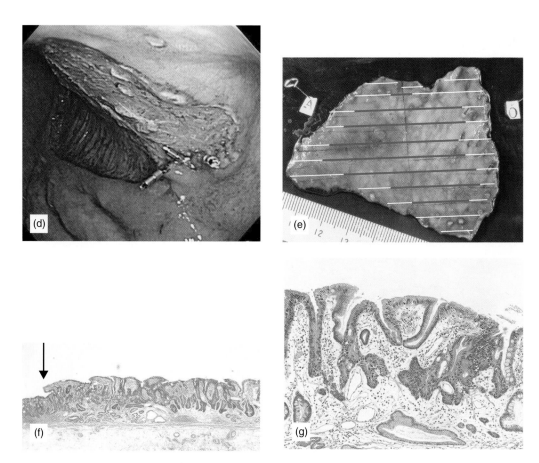

Figure 8.13 (Continued) (d) Endoscopic findings after ESD. (e) The resected specimen shows well-differentiated adenocarcinoma in the parts of red lines. A cancerous lesion exists within 5 mm from the marking spots correlating well with the extent diagnosis by magnifying endoscopy with NBI, which can confirm that the diagnosis of the extent of cancerous infiltration by the modality is accurate. Pathological findings of ESD specimen: (f) shows a flat part (0 IIb) to the right side of the black arrow and a depressed part (0 IIc) to the left, in both of which well-differentiated adenocarcinoma exists. The finding is in accordance with the histological prediction by magnifying endoscopy with NBI. (g) Type 0 IIb area is partially covered with non-neoplastic epithelium, which is the reason why the vertical margin is not clear by conventional endoscopy (Copyright M. Kaise, T. Nakayoshi, H. Tajiri).

Section 3

Colon

Optical chromoendoscopy using NBI during screening colonoscopy: its usefulness and application

9

Yasushi Sano and Shigeaki Yoshida

The detection and subsequent removal of neoplastic colorectal lesions, including adenomatous polyps and early cancers, have been reported to reduce the incidence of colorectal cancers, based on the concept of the adenoma–carcinoma sequence [1]. Therefore, the roles of screening colonoscopy and polypectomy are becoming more important because colorectal cancer is the third most common cause of cancer mortality, and the incidence of colorectal cancer in Japan is increasing [2]. Although efficacious colonoscopy is recommended, it has been reported that 10–30% of resected polyps are non-neoplastic lesions that did not need to be removed [3]. Therefore, the distinction of non-neoplastic lesions from neoplastic lesions can increase the efficiency of treatment by eliminating the time and cost of unnecessary polypectomy [4,5]. The narrowband imaging (NBI) system is based on modifying spectral features by narrowing the bandwidth of spectral transmittance with optical filters. Since 1999, we have been developing our own NBI system with support from a Grant for Scientific Research Expenses for Health and Welfare Programs, Japan. NBI modification provides a unique image emphasizing the capillary pattern (CP) and the surface structure [6–8]. In our pilot study, the NBI system was sufficient to differentiate non-neoplastic lesions from neoplastic lesions (optical chromoendoscopy), and had a special feature allowing otherwise invisible endoscopic findings to be visualized without a dye solution (high-contrast endoscopy) [8–11].

In this chapter, we describe usefulness of NBI in screening colonoscopy and target optical chromoendoscopy, and discuss the utility of the detailed observation of the micro-vascular architecture for differential diagnosis during colonoscopy.

IMPROVEMENT OF THE VISIBILITY

Our pilot study found out that, compared to the normal observation, the clearer observation of the capillary vessels in the network on the surface layer of the mucosa is possible using the NBI system [9]. Therefore, recognizing the lesion becomes easier since the permeable image of the vessels is interrupted. On the normal mucosa, regular hexagonal or honeycomb-like pattern is found around the crypt of the gland. On the other hand, in the neoplastic lesion, these vessels grow thicker and the disruption of the vessels, different diameter size of the vessels and the rise of the vessel density can be found when the abnormality gets worse. Since the filter of NBI is adjusted to hemoglobin absorption characteristics, a brownish area can be found if the observing area contains large number of capillary vessels (Figure 9.1). Contrast enhancement of the lesion made disruption of the normal vessel network in colonic lesions obvious and improved the visualization [11] (see DVD video clips 35 and 36).

IMPROVEMENT OF THE OBSERVATION OF THE SURFACE STRUCTURE (PIT PATTERN) AND THE MICRO-CAPILLARIES (CAPILLARY PATTERN)

Several studies are reporting that the observation using chromoendoscopy, and chromoendoscopy with magnifying function, is helpful for differentiating neoplasia from non-neoplasia. In our pilot study [9], the accuracy of endoscopic diagnosis was 79.1% in conventional colonoscopy and 93.4% in NBI colonoscopy. It was similar to that of chromoendoscopy with indigo carmine dye. Therefore, by combining NBI system with the magnifying function, it is expected that it is possible to infer the pit pattern on the surface layer of the mucosa without any staining and obtain as correct a diagnosis as the optical chromoendoscopy.

NBI modification provides a unique image emphasizing the CP, as well as the surface structure. Angiogenesis is critical to the transition of premalignant lesions in a hyperproliferative state to the malignant phenotype [12–14]. Therefore, the diagnosis based on the angiogenic or vascular morphological changes might be ideal for early detection or diagnosis of neoplasm. We described the utility of the detailed observation of micro-vascular architecture for differential diagnosis during NBI colonoscopy [10,15]. We have named the mucosal capillary meshwork arranged in a honeycomb pattern around the mucosal glands "meshed capillary: MC" and classified microvascular architecture using NBI colonoscopy with magnification into three types (CP, types I, II, and III) [15]. These capillary vessels which are observed clearly by NBI are thought to be similar to observing capillary vessels of around 300 μm, according to the Monte Carlo simulation that we conducted [16]. The definition of each CP is summarized in Figure 9.2 and described in detail as follows.

Normal colonic mucosa (CP: type I)

Using NBI colonoscopy without magnification, not only thick veins and thick capillaries but also fine capillaries can be seen as a brown color. The vessel network of the mucosa is well visualized in much finer detail on NBI colonoscopy compared with that on standard colonoscopy. However, the mucosal capillary meshwork (MC) arranged in a honeycomb pattern around the mucosal glands is invisible or faintly visible under magnifying observation using NBI colonoscopy (Figure 9.3(a)), because endoscopic resolution is not enough to visualize the network. The vessel diameter was reported as 8.6 ± 1.8 to $12.4 \pm 1.9 \mu m$ (range: 6.4–20.9) [13,14].

Hyperplastic polyp (CP: type I)

Most of hyperplastic polyps can be seen as light brown lesions without neovascular changes on NBI colonoscopy. Kudo's type II pit pattern can be seen by magnifying observation using NBI without any dye solution [17]. In many cases the mucosal capillary meshwork is invisible or faintly visible under magnifying observation using NBI colonoscopy, because endoscopic resolution is not enough to visualize the network (Figure 9.3(b)). We previously reported, intra-tumor micro-vessel density in small hyperplastic polyp was significantly higher than that in normal mucosa, but the vessel diameter had not significantly increased in comparison to normal mucosa [18]. However, MC vessels are sometimes recognized in a part of hyperplastic polyps such as large hyperplastic polyp [5,15] or hyperplastic polyp with serrated adenomatous change [5,15]. Still when MC vessels are seen in hyperplastic polyps they are still thin in caliber.

Adenomatous lesion (CP: type II)

Adenomatous lesion including the flat and depressed type can be seen as dark brown neovascular lesions (brownish area) on NBI colonoscopy without magnification and are easily detected while withdrawing the endoscope using NBI. Kudo's type IIIL or IV pit pattern demarcated by the appearance of MC vessels can be seen by magnifying observation using NBI without the application of any dye solution [8,15]. MC vessels can be clearly visible, because these capillaries are elongated and have increased diameters compared to the normal ones (Figure 9.3(c)). The vessel diameter is reported as $13.1 \pm 3.3\mu m$ [13,14].

Cancerous lesion (CP: type III)

Micro-vascular architecture of colonic carcinoma is characterized by a disorganized structure and increased density of micro-vessels. The vessel diameter was reported as $18.3 + 0.1$ to $19.8 + 7.6$ (range: 2.2–84.5) [13,14]. MC vessels can be clearly visible and show uneven-sized thicker capillaries with branching, curtailed appearance, and irregularity (Figure 9.3(d)). When the lesion showing "CP: type III" is identified during NBI colonoscopy, an additional detailed observation using chromoendoscopy using indigo carmine or crystal violet dye is recommended [5].

The presence of MC vessels on magnifying endoscopy using NBI is useful to distinguish between hyperplastic polyps and adenomatous polyps. Recently, we have developed the concept of detecting abnormal micro-capillaries using NBI as a marker of neoplasia from the results of our prospective study. In this study, the overall diagnostic accuracy, sensitivity, and specificity using the presence of MC vessels for distinction between neoplastic and non-neoplastic lesions were 95.3%, 96.4%, and 92.3%, respectively ($p < 0.0001$) [10]. We believe that this system speeds the assessment and simplifies the analysis of polyps as compared to real chromoendoscopy to help determine for the endoscopist whether to remove a polyp. The combination use of NBI as the initial optical chromoendoscopy and real chromoendoscopy when necessary for more advanced lesions may save time and cost on screening colonoscopy (see DVD video clip 37).

HISTOLOGICAL FINDINGS OF MICRO-VASCULAR PROLIFERATION

We evaluated micro-vascular proliferation with CD31 immunohistochemical staining in normal colonic mucosa, hyperplastic polyps, adenomas, and carcinomas (Figure 9.4). Many micro-capillary vessels measuring less than $10\mu m$ could be seen in the stroma at the surface of normal colonic mucosa and hyperplastic polyps. However, adenomatous and cancerous lesions with thicker capillary vessels ($20–30\mu m$) could be seen surrounding glands just under the basal membrane at the surface. These findings suggest that MC vessels were histologically confirmed to be dilated, with increased micro-vasculature and vessel diameters in the superficial portion of adenomatous and cancerous lesions, on immunohistochemical staining with anti-human monoclonal CD31 antibody [19].

A BENCH STUDY: COMPARISON BETWEEN ENDOSCOPIC RESOLUTION AND MC VESSELS

MC vessels in normal colonic mucosa and hyperplastic polyp are invisible or faintly visible under magnifying observation using NBI colonoscopy. To evaluate the correlation between endoscopic resolution and visibility of MC vessels, a squared plate (TOPPAN-TEST-CHART-NO1) was used in this bench study. As previously reported, MC vessels diameter are ranged 8–12 μm in normal colonic mucosa and hyperplastic polyp [12–14]. As showing in Figure 9.5(a), the approximately 8–12 μm bars on the squared plate adjusted to the same scale as the polyp could not be clearly visible or distinguishable due to the endoscopic resolution. On the other hands, MC vessels in adenomatous or cancerous lesion are ranged 13–20 μm [12–14]. These vessels are clearly visible on NBI colonoscopy with magnification (Figure 9.5(c)). In this bench study, the approximately 14–20 μm bars on the squared plate adjusted to the same scale as the polyp could be clearly visible. Therefore, the presence of MC vessels on magnifying endoscopy using NBI is a useful indicator to distinguish between hyperplastic polyps and adenomatous polyps.

ROLE AND BENEFIT OF LESION DETECTION, ASSESSMENT OF MARGINS

The data described above establish a benefit for NBI in diagnosing a polyp between adenoma and non-adenoma, and describe the theoretical basis for this. Other relevant questions regarding the use and benefit of NBI light are in the initial detection of lesions and in the assessment of margins when attempting endoscopic removal. In our initial experiments, the use of high-resolution NBI colonoscopy had a benefit for the identification of flat lesions less than 10 mm in size. The detection rate of flat lesions using high-resolution NBI colonoscopy was approximately 20% higher than that using white light colonoscopy. The effects of conventional HRE (high-resolution endoscopes) and NBI HRE on detection rates are the subjects of ongoing investigation by a number of groups.

The pit pattern observation using magnifying NBI colonoscopy is also useful for the assessment of resected margins after polypectomy or endoscopical mucosal resection. It may be necessary to perform the subsequent management such as hot biopsy or argon plasma coagulation procedure, when neoplastic pit pattern (Kudo's IIIL or IV pits) is recognized at the margin of the resected tumor.

FUTURE PROSPECTS

Diagnoses on the bases of mucosal patterns have been reported to be correlated with histological diagnoses. Chromoendoscopy is often used, as it is a contrast staining method using a biocompatible dye agent, such as indigo carmine. In mucosa with glands, the dye agents accumulate within crypt orifices. Although chromoendoscopy is effective in many applications, it is still only an optional diagnostic method because of the time consuming, additional cost, and necessity of complete mucus removal. In this review, we described the utility of detailed observation of the micro-vascular architecture for differential diagnosis during NBI colonoscopy. NBI modification provides a unique image emphasizing the CP and the surface structure. Our initial data indicate that NBI may be as effective or more effective than chromoendoscopy without having such problems [9].

Angiogenesis is critical to the transition of premalignant lesions in a hyperproliferative state to the malignant phenotype. Therefore, diagnosis based on the angiogenic or vascular morphological changes might be ideal for early detection or diagnosis of neoplasms. In this review, we have proposed the term of "MC" for distinguishing between non-neoplastic and neoplastic lesions, and the capillary classification "CP" for the differential diagnosis of colorectal lesions. On the basis of previous investigations, the surface micro-vascular architecture in colorectal lesions can be divided into three patterns: (1) honeycomb-like capillaries in the normal mucosa and hyperplastic polyps (8–12 μm), (2) elongated meshwork capillaries with of greater diameter in adenomatous lesions (~13 μm), and (3) disorganized meshwork capillaries with increased density of micro-vessels in cancerous lesions (18–19 μm) [12–14]. These CP can be easily recognized using NBI colonoscopy, and we believe that the combined use of NBI/optical chromoendoscopy and real chromoendoscopy decreases the time and cost of screening colonoscopy. The three-step strategy for the management of colorectal lesions using these procedures is shown in Figure 9.6. However, NBI colonoscopy may not be superior to chromoendoscopy for distinguishing between endoscopically treatable early invasive cancers and cancers requiring surgical management at this time. Attempts to make this determination using magnification NBI analysis of micro-vessels will require further investigation. In the meantime, we should use the three different procedures outlined in Figure 9.6 without getting them confused. A number of colon lesions are presented in Figures 9.7–9.19 as examples of the appearance of different CP's under NBI at low and high magnification with chromoendoscopic and pathologic correlation.

In the near future, we hope that NBI procedures will become standard for screening and surveillance colonoscopy. To assess the feasibility and efficacy of using the NBI system, further studies are required for colorectal lesions and other lesions of the gastrointestinal tract.

REFERENCES

1. Winawer SJ, Zauber AG, Ho MN, et al. Prevention of colorectal cancer by colonoscopic polypectomy. The National Polyp Study Workgroup. *N Engl J Med* 1993; 329(27): 1977–1981.
2. Saito H. Screening for colorectal cancer: current status in Japan. *Dis Colon Rectum* 2000; 43: S78–S84.
3. Vatan MH, Stalsbert H. The prevalence of polyps of the large intestine in Oslo: an autopsy study. *Cancer* 1982; 40: 819–825.
4. Fu KI, Sano Y, Kato S, Fujii T, Nagashima F, Yoshino T, Okuno T, Yoshida S, Fujimori T. Chromoendoscopy using indigo carmine dye spraying with magnifying observation is the most reliable method for differential diagnosis between non-neoplastic and neoplastic colorectal lesions: a prospective study. *Endoscopy* 2004; 36(12): 1089–1093.
5. Sano Y, Saito Y, Fu KI, Matsuda T, Uraoka T, Kobayashi N, Ito H, Machida H, Iwasaki J, Emura F, Hanafusa M, Yoshino T, Kato S, Fujii T. Efficacy of magnifying chromoendoscopy for the differential diagnosis of colorectal lesions. *Dig Endosc* 2005; 17(2): 105–116.
6. Sano Y, Kobayashi M, Hamamoto Y, et al. New diagnostic method based on color imaging using narrow band imaging (NBI) system for gastrointestinal tract. *Gastrointest Endosc* 2001; 53: AB125.
7. Gono K, Obi T, Yamaguchi M, Ohyama N, Machida H, Sano Y, Yoshida S, Hamamoto Y, Endo T. Appearance of enhanced tissue features in narrow-band endoscopic imaging. *J Biomed Opt* 2004; 9(3): 568–577.
8. Sano Y, Muto M, Tajiri H, Ohtsu A, Yoshida S. Optical/digital chromoendoscopy during colonoscopy using narrow band imaging system. *Dig Endosc* 2005; 17: S60–S65.
9. Machida H, Sano Y, Hamamoto Y, Muto M, Kozu T, Tajiri H, Yoshida S. Narrow band imaging for differential diagnosis of colorectal mucosal lesions: a pilot study. *Endoscopy* 2004; 36: 1094–1098.
10. Sano Y, Horimatsu T, Fu KI, et al. Magnified observation of microvascular architecture using narrow band imaging (NBI) for the differential diagnosis between non-neoplastic and neoplastic colorectal lesion: a prospective study. *Gastrointest Endosc* 2006; 63: AB102.
11. Tanaka S, Kaltenbach T, Chayama K, Soetikno R. High-magnification colonoscopy (with videos). *Gastrointest Endosc* 2006; 64(4): 604–613.
12. Konerding MA, Fait E, Gaumann A. 3D microvascular architecture of pre-cancerous lesions and invasive carcinomas of the colon. *Br J Cancer* 2001; 84(10): 1354–1362.
13. Fait E, Malkusch W, Gnoth S-H, Dimitropoulou Ch, Gaumann 2 A, Kirkpatrick CJ, Junginger Th, Konerding MA. Microvascular patterns of the human large intestine: Morphometric studies of vascular parameters in corrosion casts. *Scanning Microscopy* 1998; 12(4): 641–651.

14. Skinner SA, Frydman GM, O'Brien PE. Microvascular structure of benign and malignant tumors of the colon in humans. *Dig Dis Sci* 1995; 40(2): 373–384.
15. Sano Y, Horimatsu T, Fu KI, et al. Magnified observation of microvascular architecture of colorectal lesions using narrow band imaging system. *Dig Endosc* 2006; 18(S1): S44–S51.
16. Gono K, Yamazaki K, Doguchi N, et al. Endoscopic observation of tissue by narrowband illumination. *Opt Rev* 2003; 10: 1–5.
17. Kudo S, Hirota S, Nakajima T, et al. Colorectal tumours and pit pattern. *J Clin Pathol* 1994; 47: 880–885.
18. Sano Y, Maeda N, Kanzaki A, Fujii T, Ochiai A, Takenoshita S, Takebayashi Y. Angiogenesis in colon hyperplastic polyp. *Cancer Lett* 2005; 218(2): 223–228.
19. Muto M, Nakane M, Katada C, Sano Y, Ohtsu A, Esumi H, Ebihara S, Yoshida S. Squamous cell carcinoma in situ at oropharyngeal and hypopharyngeal mucosal sites. *Cancer* 2004; 101(6): 1375–1381.

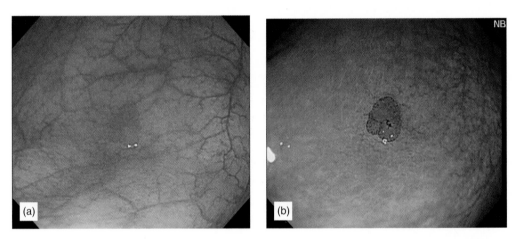

Figure 9.1 Brownish area, typical endoscopic features of flat adenomatous polyp on NBI. (a) Standard colonoscopy. 0–IIa type lesion, 4mm in size, can be seen in the rectum. (b) NBI without any dye spraying. The lesion could be seen as a dark brown lesion (brownish area) (Copyright Y. Sano, S. Yoshida).

	Schematic micro-vascular architecture	Capillary characteristics	Vessel diameter (µm) (minimum to maximum)	Visibility using NBI
Normal mucosa		Mucosal capillary network (meshwork) arranged in a honeycomb pattern around the mucosal glands.	8.6 ± 1.8 to 12.4 ± 1.9 (6.4–20.9)	MC vessel: invisible ~ faintly visible (CP: type I)
Hyperplastic		Mucosal capillary network (meshwork) arranged in a honeycomb pattern around the mucosal glands.	Usually less than 10	MC vessel: invisible ~ faintly visible (CP: type I)
Adenoma		Vascular casts showed that the micro-vasculature have a similar organization to the normal colon. However, capillaries are elongated and have increased diameters compared to normal.	13.1 ± 3.3	MC vessel: clearly visible Slightly thicker capillary Capillary density: loose (CP: type II)
Carcinoma		Vascular casts of colonic carcinoma are characterized by a disorganized structure and increased density of micro-vessels. The increased number and density of micro-vessels result in formation of nodular clusters of capillaries.	18.3 ± 0.1 to 19.8 ± 7.6 (2.2–84.5)	MC vessel: clearly visible Uneven sized thicker capillary with branching, curtailed, irregularity Capillary density: dense (CP: type III)

Figure 9.2 Sano's endoscopic micro-vascular classification of colorectal lesions using NBI (Sano's classification of CP) (Copyright Y. Sano, S. Yoshida).

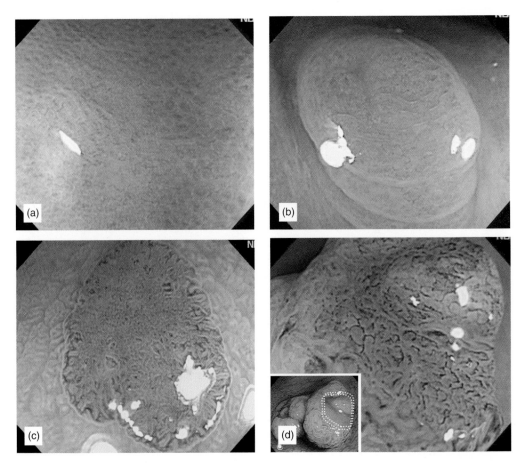

Figure 9.3 Magnifying endoscopic findings of macro-capillary vessels using NBI in normal colonic mucosa, hyperplastic polyps, adenomas, and carcinomas. (a) Normal colonic mucosa. In many cases the mucosal capillary meshwork arranged in a honeycomb pattern around the mucosal glands is invisible or faintly visible with magnifying observation using NBI colonoscopy, because the endoscopic resolution is not high enough to visualize the network (MC (−), CP: type I). (b) Hyperplastic polyps. In many cases the mucosal capillary meshwork is invisible or faintly visible with magnifying observation using NBI colonoscopy, because the endoscopic resolution is not high enough to visualize the network (MC (−), CP: type I). (c) Adenomatous polyps. MC vessels are clearly visible, because these capillaries are elongated and have longer diameters than do normal capillaries. The honeycomb-like pattern of capillaries on the surface of the tumor is retained (MC (+), CP: type II). (d) Carcinoma in adenoma (magnifying view of the demarcated area in lower-left chromoendoscopic view). The micro-vascular architecture of colonic carcinoma is characterized by a disorganized structure and increased density of micro-vessels. MC vessels are clearly visible and show unevenly sized, thicker capillaries with branching, curtailed irregularity (MC (+), CP: type III) (Copyright Y. Sano, S. Yoshida).

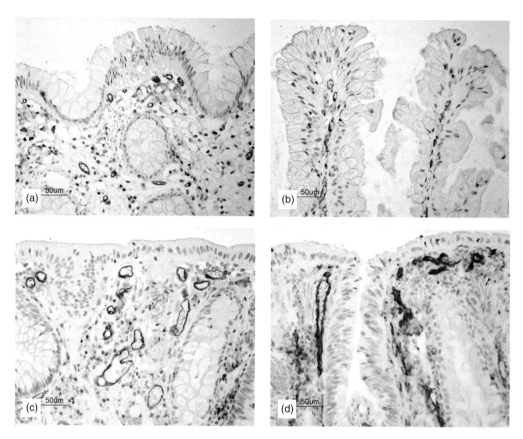

Figure 9.4 Histological findings of macro-capillary vessels in normal colonic mucosa, hyperplastic polyp, adenoma, and carcinoma. All specimens are stained for endothelial cells with an anti-CD31 antibody (clone JC/70A, DAKO, dilution 1:20). Original magnification ×100. (a) The superficial portion of normal colonic mucosa. Many micro-capillary vessels measured approximately 10 μm can be seen in the stromal tissue. (b) The superficial portion of hyperplastic polyp. Many micro-capillary vessels measured approximately 10 μm can be seen in the stromal tissue as same as normal mucosa. (c) The superficial portion of adenomatous polyp. Thicker capillary vessels can be seen surrounding the adenomatous glands. (d) The superficial portion of well-differentiated adenocarcinoma. Thicker capillary vessels can be seen surrounding the cancerous glands (Copyright Y. Sano, S. Yoshida).

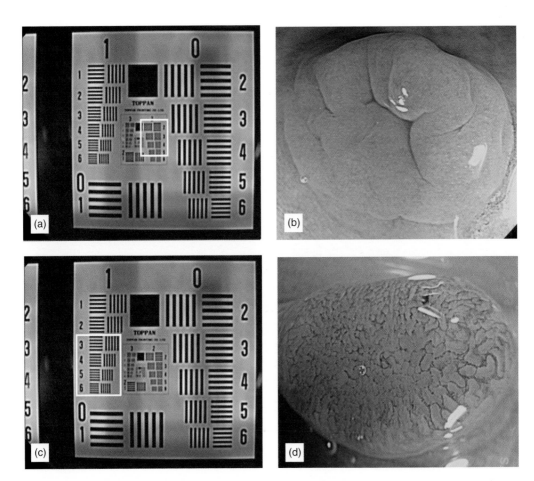

Figure 9.5 Comparison between endoscopic resolution and MC vessels. (a) Magnifying observation of squared plate (TOPPAN-TEST-CHART-NO1), 3 mm in size. The highlighted area relates
to the approximately 8–12 μm bars, which are not clearly visible or distinguishable due to the
endoscopic resolution. (b) Magnifying observation of hyperplastic polyp, also 3 mm in size,
MC (−), CP: type I. At this magnification, it is not possible to identify the MC vessels due to
8–12 μm diameter as shown in (a). (c) Magnifying observation of squared plate (TOPPAN-TEST-
CHART-NO1), 3 mm in size. The highlighted area relates to the approximately 14–20 μm bars,
which are clearly visible at this magnification. (d) Magnifying observation of adenomatous
polyp, also 3 mm in size, MC (+), CP: type II. It is possible to identify the MC vessels due to the
14–20 μm diameter as shown in (c) (Copyright Y. Sano, S. Yoshida).

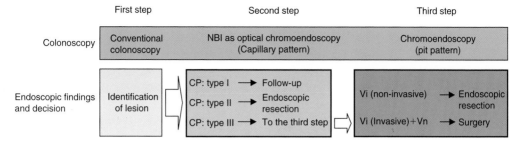

First step	Second step	Third step

	First step	Second step	Third step
Colonoscopy	Conventional colonoscopy	NBI as optical chromoendoscopy (Capillary pattern)	Chromoendoscopy (pit pattern)

| Endoscopic findings and decision | Identification of lesion | CP: type I → Follow-up
 CP: type II → Endoscopic resection
 CP: type III → To the third step | Vi (non-invasive) → Endoscopic resection
 Vi (Invasive)+Vn → Surgery |

Figure 9.6 Three-step strategy for management of colorectal lesions using conventional colonoscopy, NBI colonoscopy, and chromoendoscopy. When you find a lesion with a normal observation, observe it with NBI mode. If the result is CP type I, follow-up is recommended, CP type II, resection is recommended and CP type III, conducting chromoendoscopy, observing the pit pattern carefully, and deciding the treatment policy are recommended (Copyright Y. Sano, S. Yoshida).

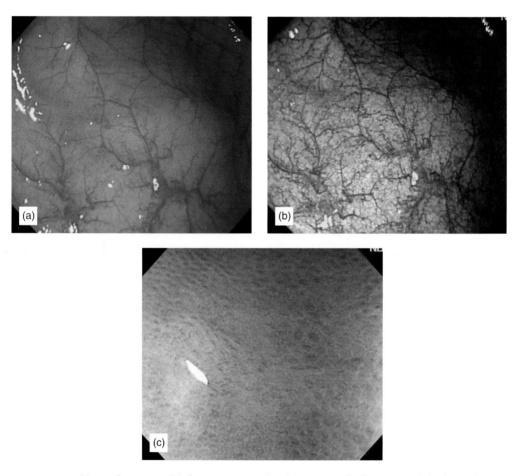

Figure 9.7 Normal mucosa. (a) On conventional colonoscopy, thick veins and thick capillaries can be seen. Using NBI, not only thick veins and thick capillaries, but also fine capillaries can be seen as a brown color. (b) NBI observation. It is possible to observe finer patterns (10 μm) compared to the normal observation. The vessel network of the mucosa is well visualized in much finer detail on NBI colonoscopy compared with that on standard colonoscopy. (c) NBI magnifying observation. It is possible to observe a type I pit pattern with magnifying observation (CP type I) (Copyright Y. Sano, S. Yoshida).

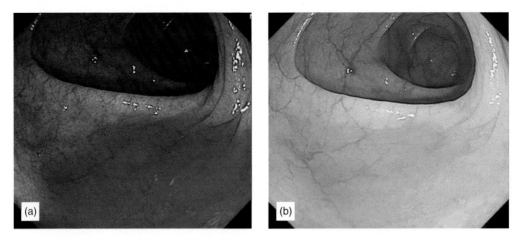

Figure 9.8 Intestinal fluids. (a) On NBI colonoscopy, intestinal fluids are recognized as reddish color fluids similar to blood. (b) This is a problem that requires improvement, because these findings give the patient an unpleasant feeling (Copyright Y. Sano, S. Yoshida).

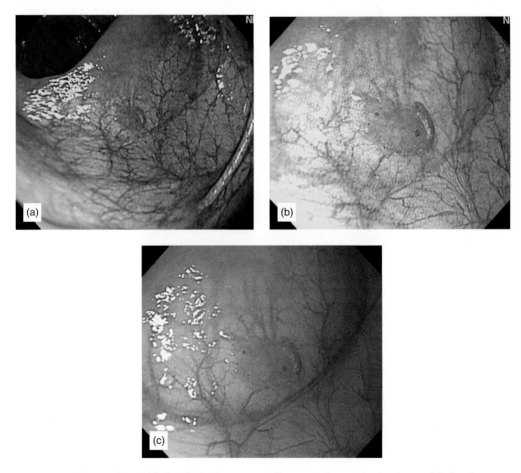

Figure 9.9 Feces. (a and b) On NBI colonoscopy, feces are also recognized as reddish color lesion similar to a reddish polyp. This is also a problem that requires improvement, because such findings are easily misinterpreted by the colonoscopist. (c) Feces on the colonic wall (Copyright Y. Sano, S. Yoshida).

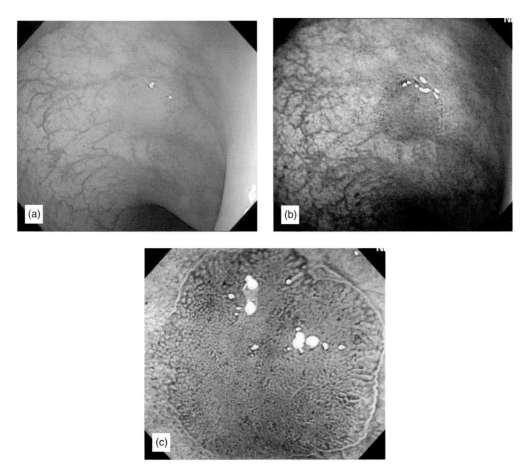

Figure 9.10 Tubular adenoma with moderate atypia, type IIa. (a) An 8-mm-sized flat elevated lesion is recognized in the area where the permeability of the capillary vessels disappears in the sigmoid colon under conventional colonoscopic observation. (b) Capillary vessels of the background mucosa become clear under NBI observation and the lesion is described as a round brown blob with improved visibility. (c) It is easy to observe IIIL + IIIs pit surrounded by MC with NBI magnifying observation (CP: type II) (Copyright Y. Sano, S. Yoshida).

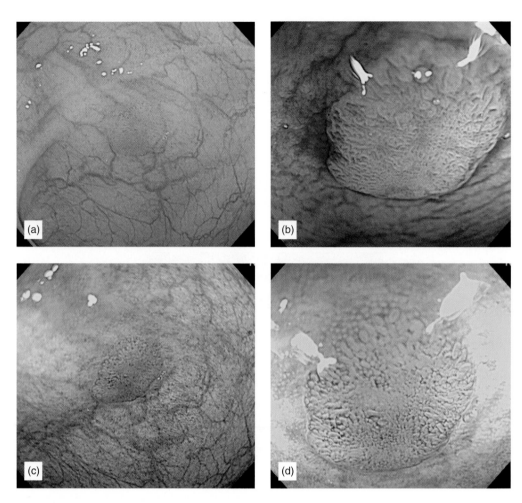

Figure 9.11 Tubular adenoma with moderate atypia, type IIa. (a) A 5-mm-sized flat polyp is recognized in the area where the permeability of the blood vessels disappears in the sigmoid colon under normal observation. (b) IIIL and IIIs pit is recognized with indigo carmine spread. (c) Capillary vessels of the background mucosa become clear under NBI observation and the lesion is described as a round brown blob with improved visibility. (d) It is easy to observe IIIL + IIIs pit surrounded by MC with NBI magnifying observation (CP: type II) (Copyright Y. Sano, S. Yoshida).

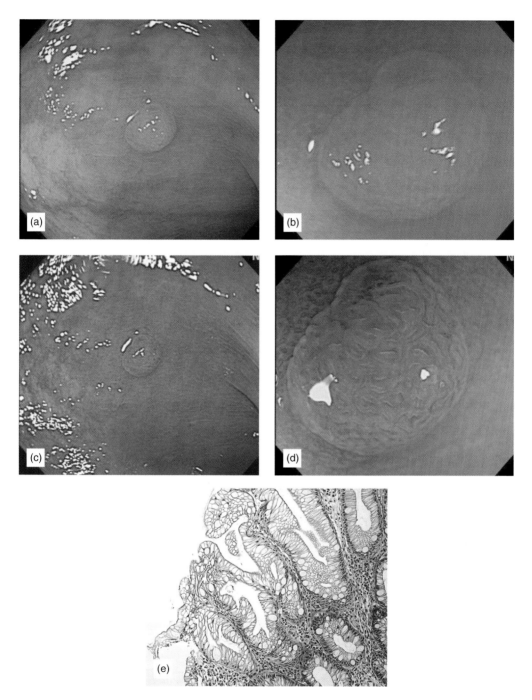

Figure 9.12 Hyperplastic polyps, type Is. (a) A 4-mm-sized sessile polyp is recognized in the sigmoid colon under normal observation. (b) Pits are unclear with a normal magnifying observation. (c and d) MC is not recognized under NBI observation and it can be diagnosed as a hyperplastic polyp (CP: type I). (e) A histopathological image. Serrated change of the duct of the gland is recognized and it is diagnosed as a hyperplastic polyp (Copyright Y. Sano, S. Yoshida).

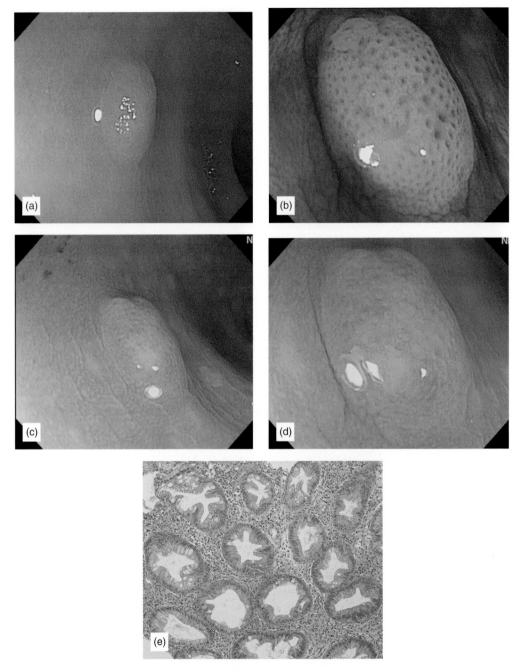

Figure 9.13 Hyperplastic polyp, type Is. (a) A faded color polyp in the sigmoid colon is recognized under the normal observation. (b) Pit pattern is recognized as type II under magnifying observation with indigo carmine spread and it is diagnosed as a hyperplastic polyp. (c and d) MC is not recognized under NBI observation and it can be diagnosed as a hyperplastic polyp (CP: type I). (e) A histopathological image. Serrated change of the duct of the gland is recognized and it is diagnosed as a hyperplastic polyp (Copyright Y. Sano, S. Yoshida).

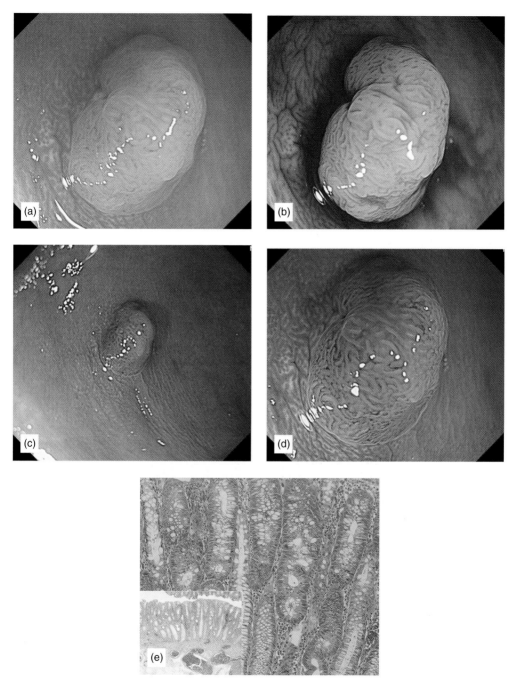

Figure 9.14 Tubular adenoma (moderately severe atypia), type Is. (a) A 7-mm-sized polyp is recognized in the sigmoid colon under normal observation. (b) Type IIIL pit pattern is recognized under magnifying observation with indigo carmine spread and it is diagnosed as an adenomatous polyp. (c and d) Under NBI observation, type IIIL pit pattern is recognized by MC which is surrounding the duct of the gland and it can be diagnosed as an adenomatous polyp (CP: type II).(e) Abnormal cells are forming abnormal ducts of the gland and the nuclear and structural atypia is both moderately severe (Copyright Y. San o, S. Yoshida).

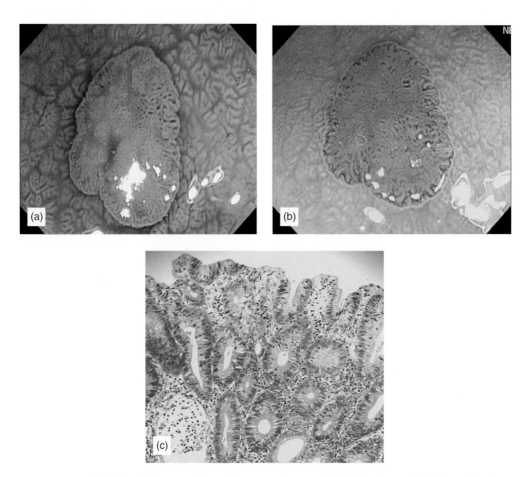

Figure 9.15 Tubular adenoma with moderate atypia, type IIa. (a) A 4-mm-sized flat polyp is recognized in the rectosigmoid. Under magnifying observation, type IIIL pit pattern is recognized under magnifying observation with indigo carmine spread and it is diagnosed as an adenomatous polyp. (b) Under NBI magnifying observation, type IIIL pit pattern is clearly recognized by MC which is surrounding the duct of the gland and it can be diagnosed as an adenomatous polyp (CP: type II). (c) Abnormal cells are forming abnormal ducts of the gland and the nuclear. The lesion is diagnosed as a tubular adenoma with moderate atypia (Copyright Y. Sano, S. Yoshida).

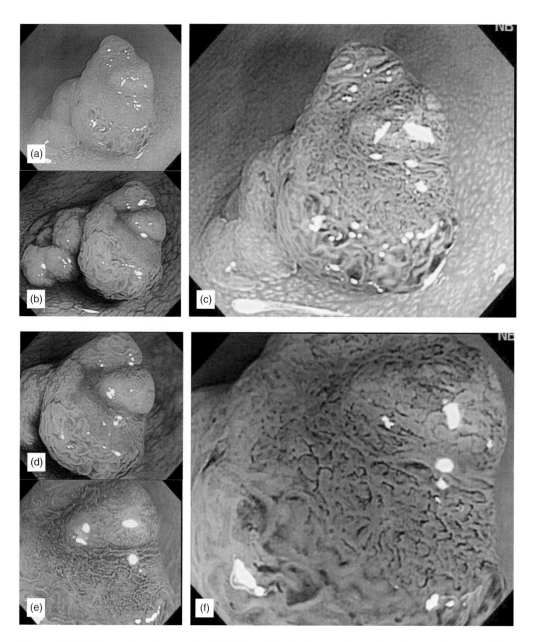

Figure 9.16 Cancer in adenoma (well-differentiated adenocarcinoma in tubular adenoma with moderate atypia), type Is. (a) A 10-mm-sized sessile polyp is recognized in the sigmoid under normal observation. Depressed surface with a small elevation is also recognized on the right side of the polyp. (b) Depressed surface on the right side becomes clearer with an indigo carmine spread magnifying observation. (c) With NBI observation, irregular capillary vessels which irregularly surround the duct of the gland on the depressed surface on the right side can be recognized (d) Indigo carmine dye with magnifying observation. Type IV pit pattern on the left side and slightly irregular type VI pit are recognized on the depressed surface on the right side. (e) Crystal violet staining image. Low-grade irregular VI pit is clearly recognized. The area of depressed surface is around 4mm and it is not diagnosed as invasive pattern but cancer in mucosa. (f) With NBI observation, irregular capillary vessels which irregularly surround the duct of the gland on the depressed surface on the right side can be recognized. And it is diagnosed as a cancer (CP: type III).

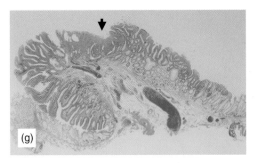

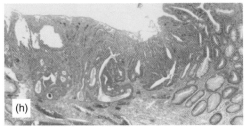

Figure 9.16 (continued) (g) EMR resection specimen. Well-differentiated adenocarcinoma in tubular adenoma with moderate atypia. Cancer is recognized on the depressed surface on the right side (see arrowhead in Figure 9.16(g). (h) Well-differentiated adenocarcinoma of the depressed surface. Muscularis mucosae is intact and the lesion is diagnosed as intramucosal cancer (Copyright Y. Sano, S. Yoshida).

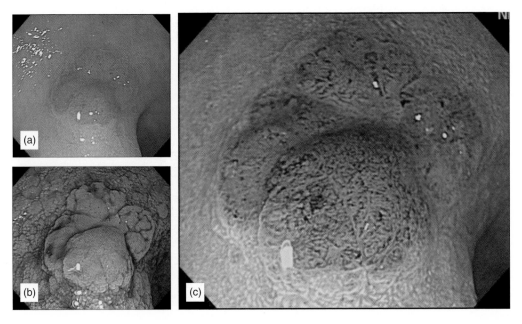

Figure 9.17 Cancer in adenoma (well-differentiated adenocarcinoma in tubular adenoma with moderate to severe atypia), type IIa (flat elevated cancer). (a) A 13-mm-sized flat elevated lesion is recognized in the rectosigmoid under normal observation. A small elevation with red flare is recognized in front middle. (b) The small elevation becomes clearer with indigo carmine spread magnifying observation. (c) With NBI observation, capillary vessels, which irregularly surround the duct of the gland in the area of a small elevation, can be recognized.

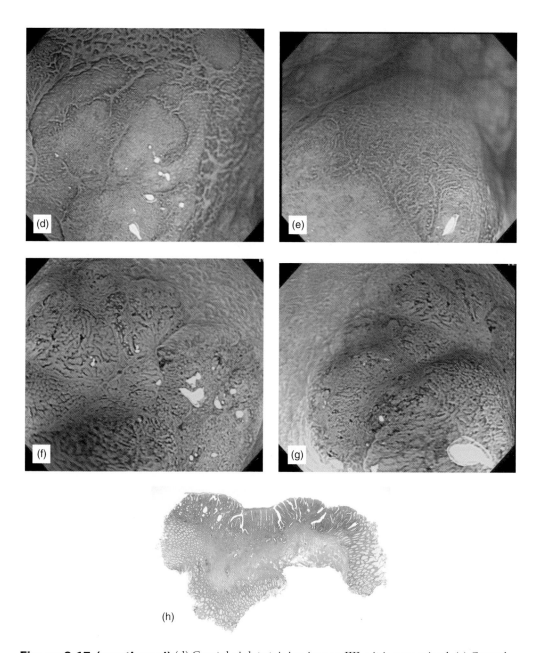

Figure 9.17 (continued) (d) Crystal violet staining image. IIIL pit is recognized. (e) Crystal violet staining image. Elevation area in front of the lesion is observed as low-grade irregular VL pit. (f) With NBI magnifying observation, fine capillary vessels with thicker diameter which surround the duct of the gland are recognized on the flat elevation area on the right side (CP: type II). (g) With NBI magnifying observation, blood vessels on the elevation in front of the lesion become thicker, presenting caliber variation and irregularly running and surrounding the duct of the gland (CP: type III). (h) EMR resection specimen. Well-differentiated adenocarcinoma in tubular adenoma with moderate to severe atypia. Depth: intramucosal cancer (Copyright Y. Sano, S. Yoshida).

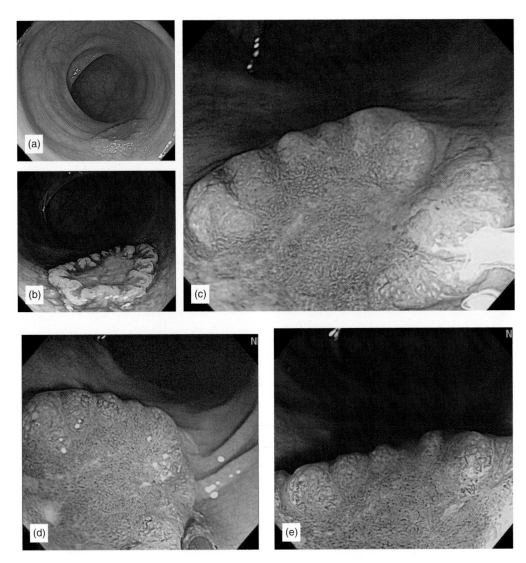

Figure 9.18 Moderately differentiated adenocarcinoma, type IIa + IIc, invasive cancer (sm1), T1. (a) A 23-mm-sized depressed lesion with white spots is recognized under normal observation. Tightened fold can be found at margins. (b) Depressed surface becomes clearer with dye magnifying observation. Star-like irregularity is recognized on the margins of the depression. (c) Crystal violet staining image. Different-sized pit with different size can be observed on the depressed surface. The structure of the pit is not destroyed and it is diagnosed as a low-grade irregular type VI pit. (d) With NBI magnifying observation, caliber variation and dense MC vessels are observed on the depressed surface (CP: type III). (e) Region of type V pit (>3mm) is recognized and it is diagnosed as the sm cancer (Copyright Y. Sano, S. Yoshida).

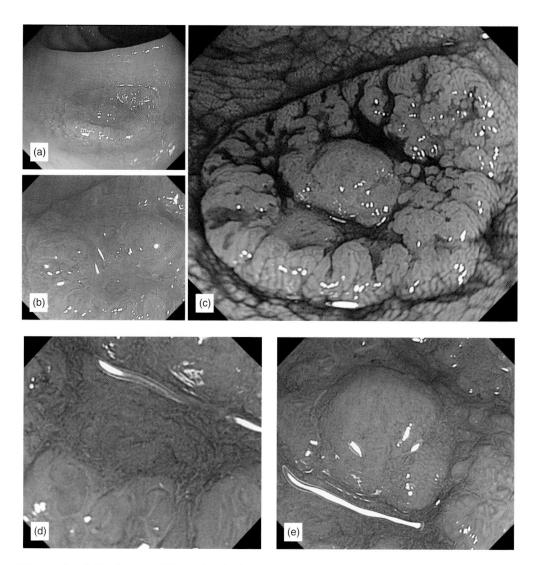

Figure 9.19 Moderately differentiated adenocarcinoma, type IIa + IIc, invasive cancer (sm1), T1. (a) A 17-mm-sized IIa + IIc depressed lesion with white spots is recognized in the rectum under normal observation. A small elevation with red flare. (b) A small elevation which presents capillary vessels with thick bore becomes clearer. (c) Indigo carmine spread image. Star-like irregularity is recognized at margins of the depression. Pit in a different size which is arranged on the depressed surface of the lesion of front left side. The structure of the pit is not destroyed and it is diagnosed as low-grade irregular type VI pit. (d). Crystal violet staining image. Magnifying observation of the left below part of the lesion. Unsteady high-grade irregular type VI pit is observed in whirlpool shape. (e) Crystal violet staining image. Magnifying observation of the middle part of the lesion. Low-grade irregular type VI pit is observed.

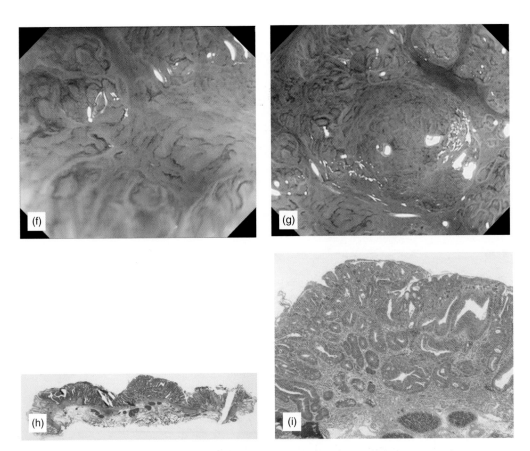

Figure 9.19 (continued) (f) NBI magnifying observation of the region of the above (d). Irregular disruption and meander is observed (CP: type III). (g) NBI magnifying observation of the region of the above (e). Tumor blood vessels with different size of bore which run irregularly are recognized. It is determined to be a blood vessels image of cancer (CP: type III). (h and I) Moderately differentiated adenocarcinoma is recognized. Sm infiltration is found in the elevation area of the depressed area which is recognized by an endoscope (infiltration distance 375 m). It was reported as ly0 and V0 (Copyright Y. Sano, S. Yoshida).

The significance of NBI observation for inflammatory bowel diseases

10

Takayuki Matsumoto, Tetsuji Kudo and Mitsuo Iida

NBI (narrowband imaging) is characterized by a light source that produces narrowband and spectroscopically characteristic light. NBI is the technology which enhances specific depth and color tone. By means of the NBI system with narrow band filter that has the absorption property of hemoglobin, vascular architecture and surface structure as outlined by vessels in the gastrointestinal mucosa are enhanced. As a result, NBI is a useful procedure for the detection of neoplasms and the diagnosis of tumor depth in the gastrointestinal tract.

We applied NBI colonoscopy for patients with chronic colon inflammatory bowel disease. The instruments we used were CLV-260SL as a NBI light source and video processor CV-260SL. We used CF-H260AI colonoscopies produced by Olympus Corporation for NBI observation.

Comparisons of images of colonic ulcers among conventional colonoscopy, NBI, and chromoendoscopy with indigo carmine are illustrated in Figure 10.1. In NBI, vascular-like structures are observed clearly and crypt openings in the reddish mucosa around the ulcer are enhanced. On the other hand, the elevated or depressed areas become obvious by chromoendoscopy, even though the vascular pattern is obscure.

ULCERATIVE COLITIS

Determination of endoscopic severity

In active ulcerative colitis (UC), conventional colonoscopy discerns disappearance of mucosal vascular pattern (MVP), fine or coarse granular mucosa, mucous exudates and mucosal defects. In quiescent UC, distorted MVP, inflammatory polyps, and scarred ulcers are observed. In some occasions, the conventional colonoscopic findings completely normalize. Because

NBI is a procedure suitable for the observation of vasculature, MVP is the best target for NBI observation in UC to determine the severity.

In addition, the histological severity may be assessed, and furthermore, subsequent response to therapy may be predicted when NBI is coupled with magnifying endoscopy. According to Fujiya and colleagues, minute defects of epithelium, mucus exudates, and villous- or coral reef-like mucosa are characteristic magnifying colonoscopic findings in histologically active UC [1]. Among those findings, coral reef-like mucosa, which is presumed to conform to invisible network pattern without crypt openings in our classification, seems to be the most significant finding, which indicates histologically active disease. It thus seems probable that villous- or coral reef-like mucosa and crypt openings are findings, which need to be identified clearly by NBI in UC.

Active UC

Small yellowish spots (Figures 10.2 and 10.3) and mucus exudates (Figures 10.4 and 10.5) under conventional colonoscopy are observed as localized white spots under NBI. On the other hand, actively inflamed mucosa, which is marked by disappearance of MVP, fine granular mucosa, and spontaneous bleeding under conventional colonoscopy, is depicted as brownish mucosa in NBI observation. NBI in active UC occasionally depicts vessels in the deep layer, which cannot be observed by conventional colonoscopy (Figures 10.4 and 10.5). These vessels in the deep layer, which appear commonly in NBI under normal conditions as linear, green structures, are generally obscure in active UC (Figures 10.4–10.6). When an observation with appropriate distance from the mucosa is applied, NBI can detect patchy and skipped involvement that is found in approximately 30% of patients with active UC (Figure 10.7).

By means of NBI observation, circular pits of crypt openings and mucosal surface patterns, which conform to either coral reef-like appearance (Figures 10.4 and 10.5) or villous appearance (Figure 10.6), can be easily observed in active UC. However, there is a need for the assessment of round pits under both white light and NBI, because crypt openings cannot be distinguished from yellowish spots by the procedure alone. While conventional colonoscopy is superior to NBI for the determination of small yellowish spots (Figures 10.2 and 10.3), crypt openings are better emphasized by NBI (Figures 10.4–10.6).

Quiescent UC

As has been described above, NBI is useful for the assessment of MVP. This is especially the case for quiescent UC. The MVP under NBI comprises two distinctive patterns: one being a deep vasculature appearing green in color and the other superficial vasculature that is brown in color.

When UC has completely healed, conventional colonoscopy depicts MVP as seen in normal subjects. On that occasion, both green vessels in the deep layer and brownish vessels in the more superficial layer are observed clearly by NBI (Figures 10.8 and 10.9). By simultaneous application of magnifying observation, the small and regular vascular network in the superficial layer can be depicted more clearly. However, MVP in the superficial layer may become obscure under NBI observation in the mucosa with slightly distorted MVP (Figure 10.10).

On the other hand, the pattern of MVP is divided into two types, when quiescent UC with pale mucosa is observed by NBI colonoscopy. In one pattern, the superficial brown vessels are enhanced (Figures 10.11 and 10.12) and in the other pattern the brownish vessels become obscure with obvious crypt openings (Figures 10.13–10.15). When compared with histological findings, the obscure brown vessel pattern tended to represent more severe inflammatory infiltrates, and more frequent goblet cell depletion and basal plasmacytosis. It thus seems to be reasonable to evaluate superficial MVP by NBI colonoscopy in quiescent UC.

Diagnosis of dysplasia

Because patients with UC are at high risk for the development of colorectal cancer, endoscopic surveillance is a recommended strategy for the disease. In recent years, it has been confirmed that target biopsy with chromoendoscopy and magnifying colonoscopy is useful for the detection of neoplastic lesions during surveillance colonoscopy. As has been demonstrated previously, chromoendoscopy is a procedure to identify protruding or depressed lesions and magnifying colonoscopy to identify pit pattern specific to neoplastic lesions [2].

NBI colonoscopy is a procedure to enhance vessels and the corresponding pit pattern, rather than to enhance the height of the mucosa. Thus, the major value of NBI colonoscopy for the case of surveillance colonoscopy in UC is to confirm in a suspected raised or depressed lesion the presence of a pit pattern specific to neoplasia. It is thus presumed that the site for target biopsy can be identified from among the large colorectal area by the pit pattern under NBI without chromoendoscopy. Although it remains to be elucidated, there is also another possibility that the vascular pattern per se determined by NBI may be different between inflammation and dysplasia, allowing for the detection or diagnosis of dysplasia in mucosa that is not grossly polypoid.

Figure 10.16 shows dysplasia in a patient with UC, which was found by NBI. Although the lesion was not discerned by conventional colonoscopy, a diminutive localized lesion with IIIL pit pattern was detected by NBI observation. Biopsy specimen obtained from the lesion contained high-grade dysplasia. As has been illustrated in the case, it seems possible that NBI may be a useful tool in surveillance colonoscopy and more convenient when compared to chromoendoscopy for this purpose. In order to improve the diagnostic value of NBI in this field, it seems that further investigation will be necessary to elucidate more precisely the pit patterns of dysplasia in UC.

CROHN'S DISEASE

In addition to major intestinal manifestations such as cobblestone appearance of the intestine and longitudinal ulcers, patients with Crohn's disease (CD) manifest small, aphthoid ulcers within the gastrointestinal tract.

In cases of CD, we could not confirm any practical significance of NBI for the observation of major disease involvement; much of this is readily apparent under white light examination. In contrast, NBI observation was useful for the identification of aphthoid ulcer and lymphoid hyperplasia, which coexisted frequently in patents with CD. As indicated in Figures 10.17 and 10.18, a small elevation with central depression, which was not depicted by conventional colonoscopy, became evident by means of NBI colonoscopy.

To date, we have not had any cases of dysplasia in CD that have undergone examination by magnification NBI. We cannot therefore make any comment yet on particular findings or patterns in NBI for dysplastic colonic mucosa in patients with Crohn's.

CONCLUSION

It seems to be unequivocal that NBI colonoscopy contributes to the improvement of the screening examination for and precise diagnosis of colorectal neoplasms. As has been described in this chapter, NBI observation seems to provide important information for the assessment of pathophysiology in patients with chronic inflammatory bowel disease. This seems to be especially the case for the evaluation of MVP in UC, which has not been systematically and objectively scored by conventional colonoscopy. In addition, NBI seems to contribute to the detection and diagnosis of dysplasia in these patients (see DVD video clips 47–49).

REFERENCES

1. Fujiya M, Saitoh Y, Nomura M, et al. Minute findings by magnifying colonoscopy are useful for the evaluation of ulcerative colitis. *Gastrointest Endosc* 2002; 56: 535–542.
2. Kudo S, Tamura S, Nakajima T, et al. Diagnosis of colorectal tumorous lesions by magnifying colonoscopy. *Gastrointest Endosc* 1996; 44: 8–14.

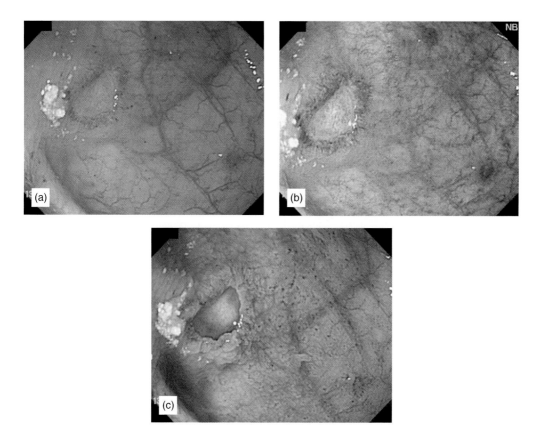

Figure 10.1 Comparisons of the images for a colonic ulcer obtained by conventional colonoscopy, NBI colonoscopy, and chromoendoscopy with indigo carmine solution. (a) Under conventional colonoscopy, an ulcer and the surrounding reddish mucosa can be seen. (b) Under NBI colonoscopy, superficial vascular network around the ulcer is clearly depicted in brownish color. Vessels in the deep layer are observed in green. The red area indicates residual feces. (c) Chromoendoscopy shows the margin of the ulcer more clearly. Crypt openings in flat mucosa are also discerned. However, MVP cannot be seen (Copyright T. Matsumoto, T. Kudo, M. Iida).

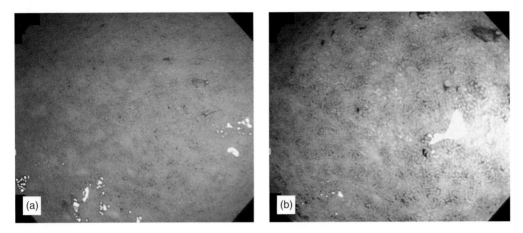

Figure 10.2 Mildly active UC. (a) Observation under conventional colonoscopy. (b) By NBI observation, crypt openings enlarged to villous-like structure is clearly observed. Deep, green-colored vessels can be seen (Copyright T. Matsumoto, T. Kudo, M. Iida).

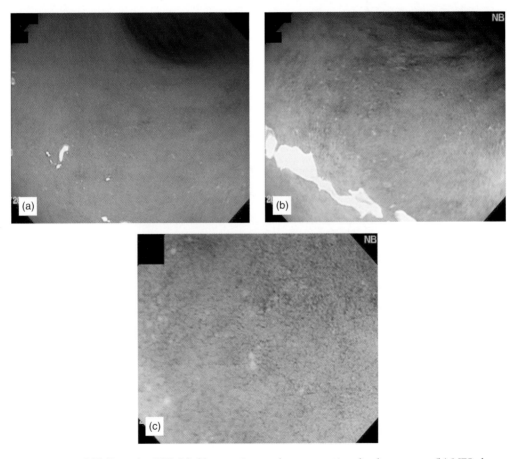

Figure 10.3 Mildly active UC. (a) Observation under conventional colonoscopy. (b) NBI observation. (c) NBI observation with magnifying colonoscopy. White spots and crypt openings are clearly depicted. However, MVP vessel cannot be observed (Copyright T. Matsumoto, T. Kudo, M. Iida).

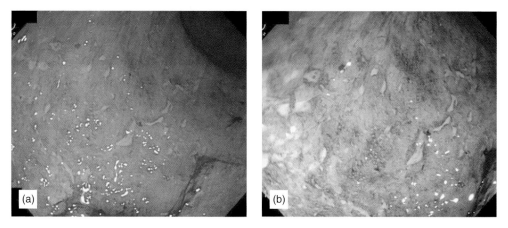

Figure 10.4 Moderately active UC. (a) Observation under conventional colonoscopy. (b) In NBI observation, mucus exudates are depicted as whitish area. Coral reef-like mucosa is evident (Copyright T. Matsumoto, T. Kudo, M. Iida).

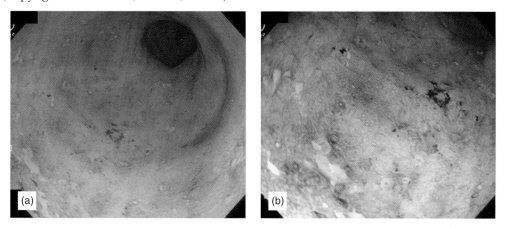

Figure 10.5 Mildly active UC. (a) Observation under conventional colonoscopy. (b) Even in NBI observation, vessels cannot be observed. There is coral reef-like mucosa (Copyright T. Matsumoto, T. Kudo, M. Iida).

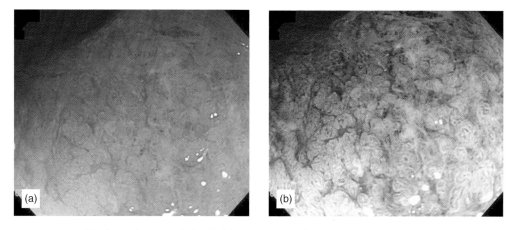

Figure 10.6 Moderately active UC. (a) Observation under conventional colonoscopy. (b) In NBI observation, small intestinal villous structure becomes clear (Copyright T. Matsumoto, T. Kudo, M. Iida).

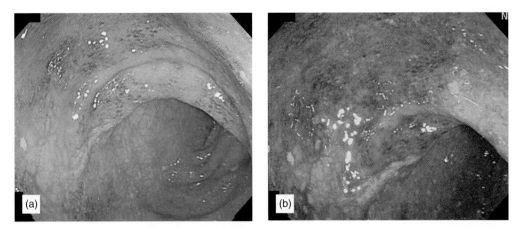

Figure 10.7 Skipped involvement. (a) Observation under conventional colonoscopy. (b) In NBI observation, discontinuous lesion can be observed as a brownish area (Copyright T. Matsumoto, T. Kudo, M. Iida).

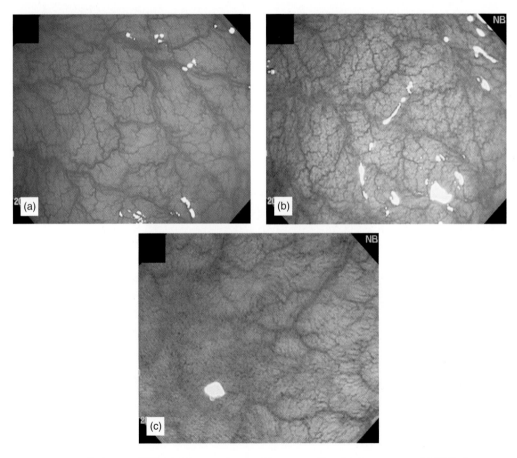

Figure 10.8 Quiescent UC. (a) Observation under conventional colonoscopy. (b) NBI observation. (c) NBI observation with magnifying colonoscopy. In NBI, it is possible to clarify deep green vessels and brownish superficial vessels. Magnifying observation shows vessels and crypt openings clearly (Copyright T. Matsumoto, T. Kudo, M. Iida).

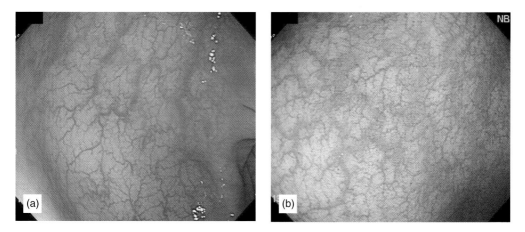

Figure 10.9 Quiescent UC. (a) Observation under conventional colonoscopy. (b) NBI observation shows clear MVP (Copyright T. Matsumoto, T. Kudo, M. Iida).

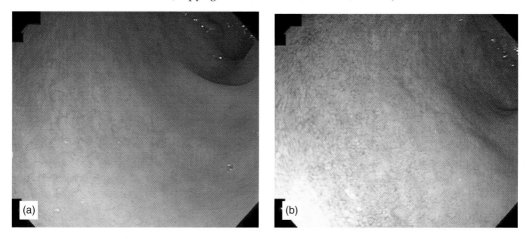

Figure 10.10 Quiescent UC. (a) Observation under conventional colonoscopy. (b) NBI observation shows deep vessels. However, superficial vessels are not discerned (Copyright T. Matsumoto, T. Kudo, M. Iida).

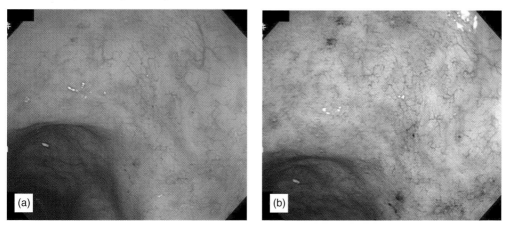

Figure 10.11 Quiescent UC. (a) Observation under conventional colonoscopy. (b) In NBI observation, deep vessels and tortuous superficial vessels can be seen (Copyright T. Matsumoto, T. Kudo, M. Iida).

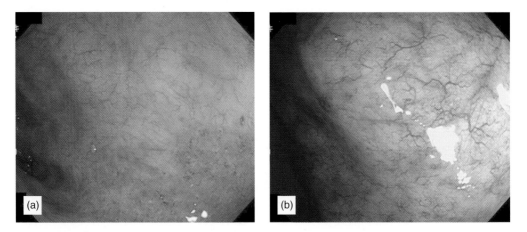

Figure 10.12 Quiescent UC. (a) Observation under conventional colonoscopy. (b) In NBI observation, superficial vessels can be clearly observed (Copyright T. Matsumoto, T. Kudo, M. Iida).

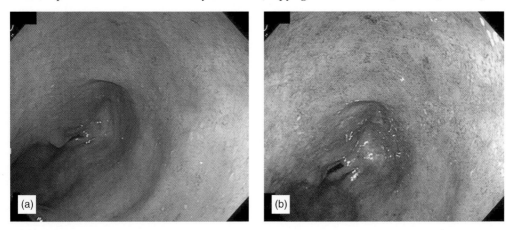

Figure 10.13 Quiescent UC. (a) Observation under conventional colonoscopy. (b) NBI observation. Although deep vessels can be seen, superficial vessels are obscure (Copyright T. Matsumoto, T. Kudo, M. Iida).

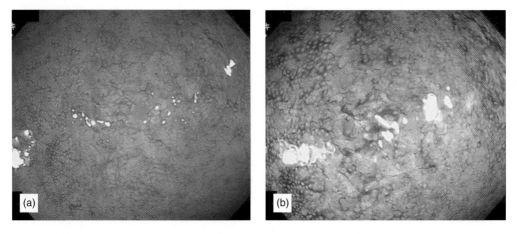

Figure 10.14 Quiescent UC. (a) Observation under conventional colonoscopy. (b) In NBI observation, crypt openings, rather than superficial vessels, are clear (Copyright T. Matsumoto, T. Kudo, M. Iida).

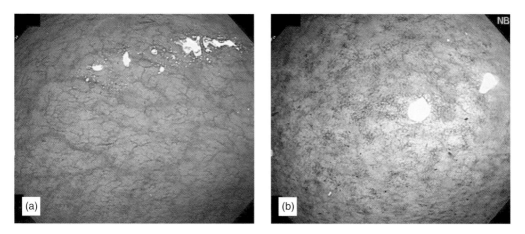

Figure 10.15 Quiescent UC. (a) Observation under conventional colonoscopy. (b) NBI observation. Although deep vessels can be seen, superficial vessels are obscure (Copyright T. Matsumoto, T. Kudo, M. Iida).

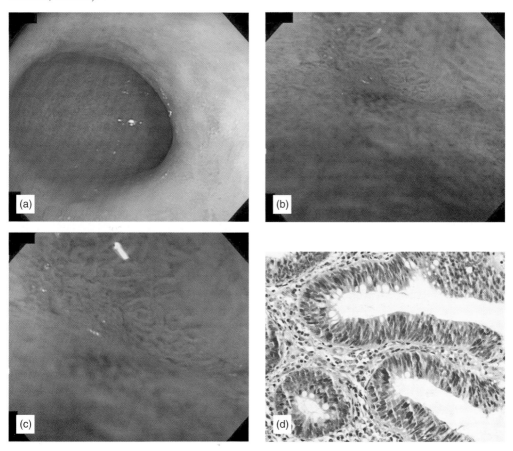

Figure 10.16 A case of high-grade dysplasia in UC. (a) No lesion can be discerned under conventional colonoscopy. (b) In NBI observation, there is an area of IIIL pit pattern, which is distinctive of the surrounding mucosa. (c) Magnifying observation shows the area to be composed of IIIL and IIIs pit patterns. (d) Histology of the biopsy specimen shows high-grade dysplasia (Copyright T. Matsumoto, T. Kudo, M. Iida).

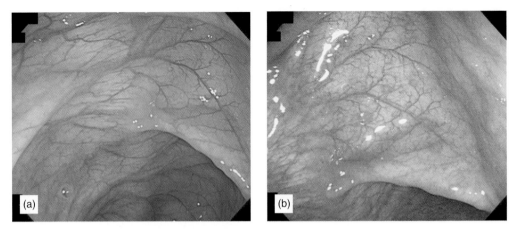

Figure 10.17 Colonoscopic findings in a case of CD of ileitis. (a) Observation under conventional colonoscopy. (b) In NBI observation, lymphoid hyperplasia becomes evident (Copyright T. Matsumoto, T. Kudo, M. Iida).

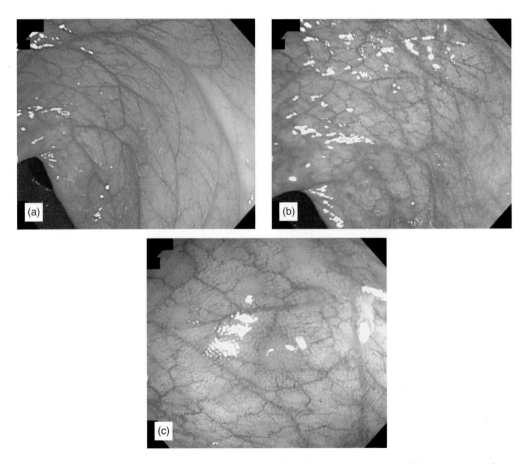

Figure 10.18 Colonoscopic findings in a case of CD of aphthous type. (a) Observation under conventional colonoscopy. (b) NBI observation. (c) Close-up view under NBI. Lymphoid hyperplasia is seen clearly (Copyright T. Matsumoto, T. Kudo, M. Iida).

Part III

Atlas of Images and Histopathologic Correlates

Pharynx and esophagus atlas

11

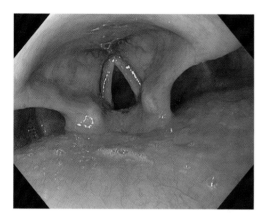

Figure 11.1 High resolution white light image of normal vocal cords (NYU School of Medicine).

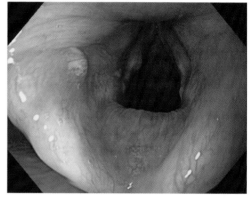

Figure 11.2 Small nodule on arytenoid and cyst on vocal cord (Erasmus University Hospital).

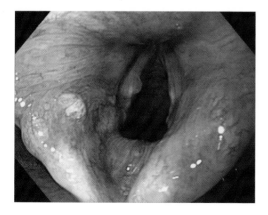

Figure 11.3 Small nodule on arytenoid and cyst on vocal cord seen more easily on NBI low-magnification view (Erasmus University Hospital).

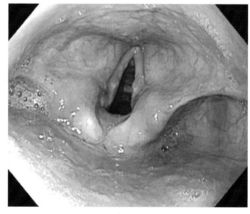

Figure 11.4 This white light HRE clearly shows erythema of the aryepligottic folds in this patient with endoscopically confirmed active GERD and throat clearing (NYU School of Medicine).

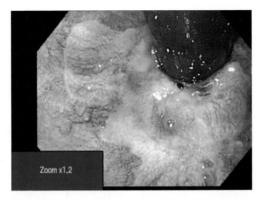

Figure 11.5 Turnaround view highlights normal stratified squamous mucosa of the distal esophagus well delineated on NBI magnification view (Institute Arnault Tzanck).

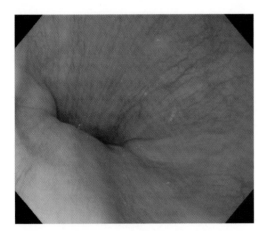

Figure 11.6 Palisade vessels in normal esophageal mucosa, important to the localization of the top of the gastric folds (Catholic University of the Sacred Heart).

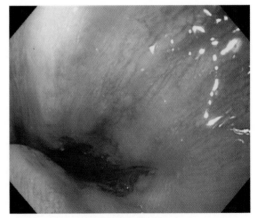

Figure 11.7 NBI view of palisade vessels in normal distal esophageal mucosa (Catholic University of the Sacred Heart).

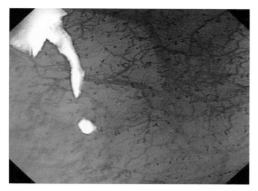

Figure 11.8 Type I intra-epithelial papillary capillary loops (IPCL) seen under NBI low magnification view of normal esophageal mucosa. These appear here as characteristic brown dots in a "pinhair" pattern (Showa University Northern Yokohama Hospital) (Copyright H. Inoue).

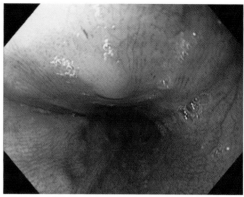

Figure 11.9 Normal esophagus in NBI view with normal IPCL pattern to the left of the image and no visible IPCL pattern to the right (Erasmus University Hospital).

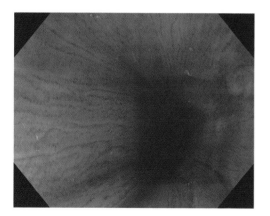

Figure 11.10 Normal esophageal stratified squamous epithelium IPCL pinhair pattern seen as brown dots, NBI 1.5 × magnification (NYU School of Medicine).

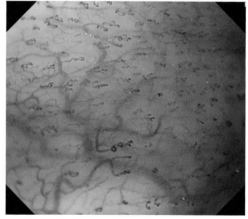

Figure 11.11 Normal brown IPCL pattern with deeper green branching vessels below (National Cancer Center Hospital East) (Copyright M. Muto).

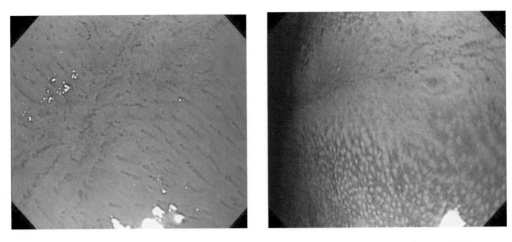

Figure 11.12 Type 2 IPCL-GERD. Enlarged but regularly arranged IPCL is observed. (Showa University Northern Yokohama Hospital) (Copyright H. Inoue).

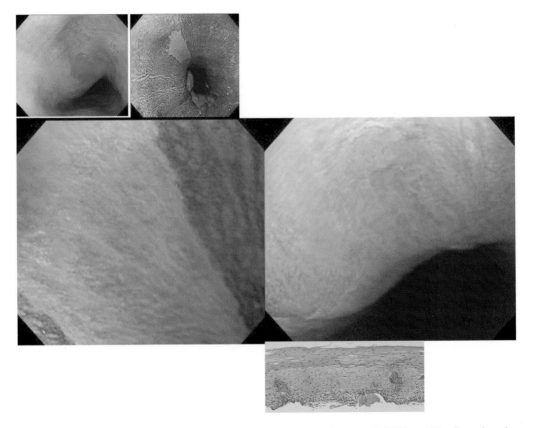

Figure 11.13 IPCL Type III pattern present is chronic esophagitis. IPCL Type III reflects lugol-void area with no IPCL proliferation. The magnification view of the capillary pattern shows that this is a benign lesion despite the non-staining with iodine similar to squamous cell carcinoma (Showa University Northern Yokohama Hospital) (Copyright H. Inoue).

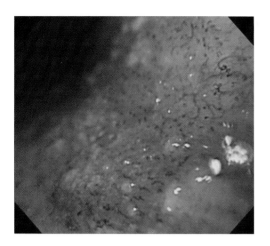

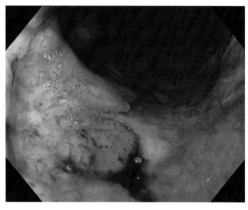

Figure 11.14 Type IV IPCL seen on magnification NBI. IPCL Type IV reflects an area with IPCL proliferation. (Showa University Northern Yokohama Hospital) (Copyright H. Inoue).

Figure 11.15 Irregular vessels in squamous CA, close up with HRE and NBI without zoom (University Medical Center Hamburg Eppendorf).

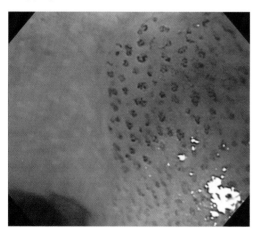

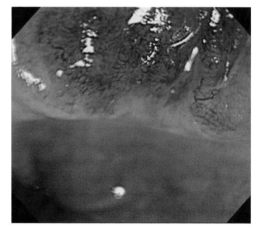

Figure 11.16 Type V-1 IPCL seen on magnification NBI in a superficial squamous carcinoma. IPCL Type V-1 reflects an area with marked IPCL proliferation and meandering of it. Note the combination of irregular high density and thicker vessels with a sharp demarcation in this flat cancer (Showa University Northern Yokohama Hospital) (Copyright H. Inoue).

Figure 11.17 NBI magnification view of invasive SCC as manifest by neovessel IPCL (Type Vn) (Showa University Northern Yokohama Hospital) (Copyright H. Inoue).

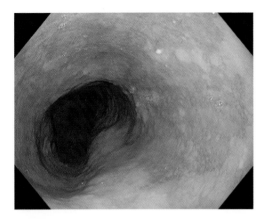

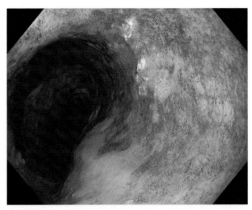

Figure 11.18 Esophageal mucosal squamous cell carcinoma (SCC), HRE low magnification view. This appears on white light as a flat reddened area and might be mistaken for an inlet patch of ectopic gastric mucosa (see Figures 11.21–11.23) without better examination of the mucosal surface and vascular pattern with NBI and magnification (Mayo Clinic, Jacksonville).

Figure 11.19 Esophageal mucosal NBI low-magnification view of esophageal SCC. Magnification required to really assess the vascular pattern. Dense dark vessels and irregular surface are evident, as well as demarcation from normal tissue (Mayo Clinic, Jacksonville).

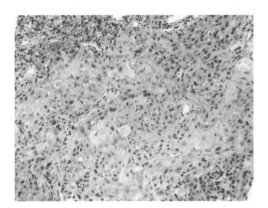

Figure 11.20 Histologic image demonstrating SCC (corresponds to Figures 11.18 and 11.19) (Mayo Clinic, Jacksonville).

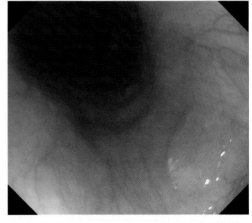

Figure 11.21 This small proximal reddish lesion may raise a concern for esophageal SCC (corresponds to Figures 11.22–11.23) (National Cancer Center Hospital East) (Copyright M. Muto).

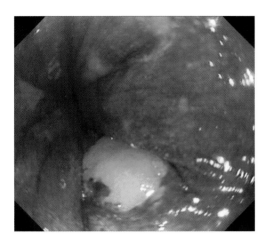

Figure 11.22 Ectopic gastric mucosa which still does not stain by iodine solution, similar to a SCC (corresponds to Figures 11.21 and 11.23) (National Cancer Center Hospital East) (Copyright M. Muto).

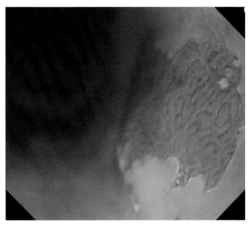

Figure 11.23 Magnification NBI image shows regular gastric mucosal pattern with no abnormal brown IPCLs that would be present in an SCC (National Cancer Center Hospital East) (Copyright M. Muto).

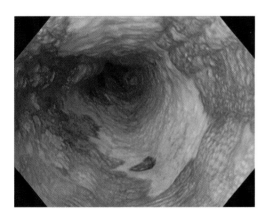

Figure 11.24 Flat squamous CA Lugol staining under white light HRE. The margin of the lesion is distinguished easily (University Medical Center Hamburg Eppendorf).

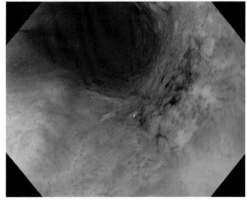

Figure 11.25 HRE NBI image corresponding to Lugol staining. NBI adds the vascular pattern and still allows to distinguish margins (University Medical Center Hamburg Eppendorf).

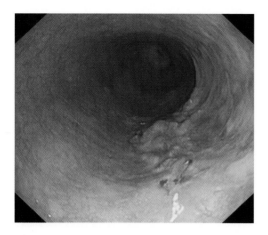

Figure 11.26 White light magnified view of squamous cell esophageal carcinoma. Histology revealed an invasive well-differentiated SCC (University of Amsterdam).

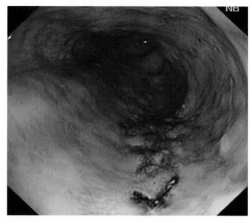

Figure 11.27 NBI image of this lesion prior to Lugol staining delineates margins well (University of Amsterdam).

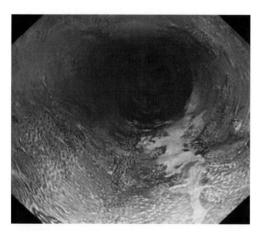

Figure 11.28 Lugol stain shows similar outline of tumor extent to the NBI image (University of Amsterdam).

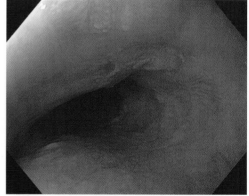

Figure 11.29 SCC on white HRE view detected as slightly depressed, erythroplastic area (corresponds to Figures 11.30–11.32) (Edouard Herriot Hospital).

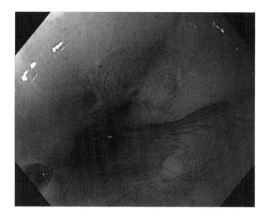

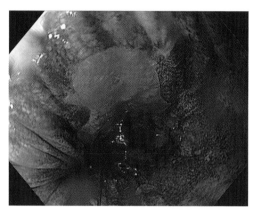

Figure 11.30 Slightly depressed SCC: red-brown on NBI (because of hypervascularization). Note the sharp demarcation and the irregular IPCL pattern (corresponds to Figures 11.29, 11.31 and 11.32) (Edouard Herriot Hospital).

Figure 11.31 Slightly depressed SCC: Lugol image provides similar information to the NBI view (Edouard Herriot Hospital).

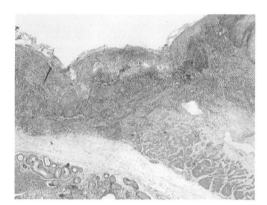

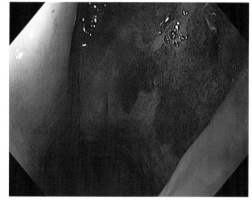

Figure 11.32 Squamous carcinoma invades the mucosa and superficial submucosa (corresponds to Figures 11.29–11.31) (Edouard Herriot Hospital).

Figure 11.33 Lower limit of a superficial SCC: good delineation of the extent of the lesion with NBI (corresponds to Figure 11.34) (Edouard Herriot Hospital).

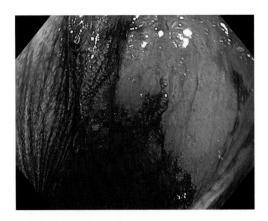

Figure 11.34 Lower limit of a superficial SCC: Lugol staining provides the same information as NBI in this case (corresponds to Figure 11.33) (Edouard Herriot Hospital).

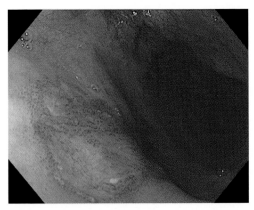

Figure 11.35 NBI image reveals two lesions of superficial SCC. The abnormal IPCL pattern is evident on the proximal lesion (Edouard Herriot Hospital).

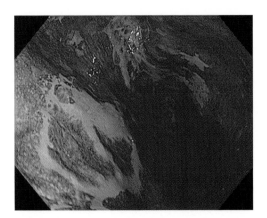

Figure 11.36 These same two lesions of superficial SCC: Lugol (same pattern as with NBI). When iodine is used, non-staining area should be watched for transition into pink color indicative of carcinoma (corresponds to Figure 11.35) (Edouard Herriot Hospital).

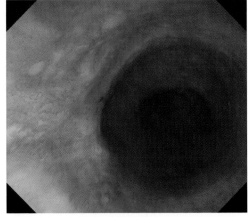

Figure 11.37 White light view of a superficial squamous cell carcinoma of the esophagus notable for non-specific discoloration and bumpy surface appearance (corresponds to Figures 11.38 and 11.39) (National Cancer Center Hospital East) (Copyright M. Muto).

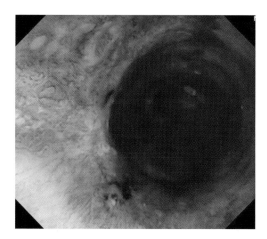

Figure 11.38 NBI nicely delineates the margin of this SCC occupying a wide proportion of the circumference of the esophagus (corresponds to Figures 11.37 and 11.39) (National Cancer Center Hospital East) (Copyright M. Muto).

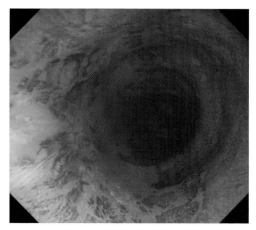

Figure 11.39 SCC. In this case, Lugols provides similar information to NBI view in terms of margin (National Cancer Center Hospital East) (Copyright M. Muto).

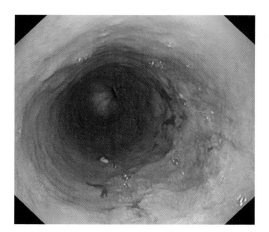

Figure 11.40 This low-magnification image of a SCC in white light HRE shows reddened area with raised contours and is easily recognized as abnormal (University of Amsterdam).

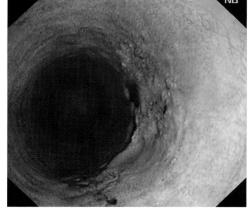

Figure 11.41 NBI low-magnification image clearly visualizes abnormality (corresponds to Figures 11.40 and 11.42 (University of Amsterdam).

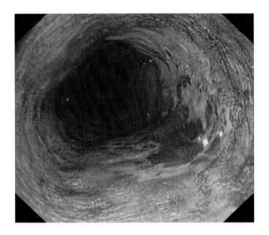

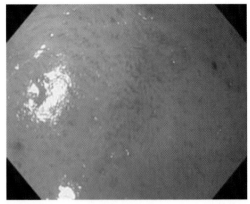

Figure 11.42 Lugol stain in this case better delineates the margins of the superficial carcinoma than NBI image (corresponds to Figures 11.40 and 11.41) (University of Amsterdam).

Figure 11.43 Small-discolored lesion seen on white light found to be a (3 × 7 mm) triangular squamous carcinoma on EMR specimen (Edouard Herriot Hospital).

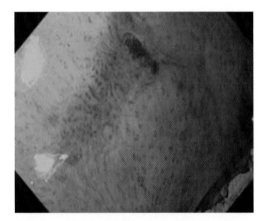

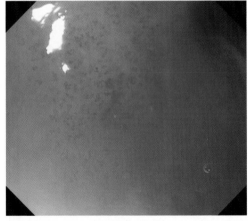

Figure 11.44 Better delineation of extent of this lesion possible with NBI, low-magnification view (corresponds to Figure 14.43) (Edouard Herriot Hospital).

Figure 11.45 Hypopharynx, left pyriform sinus, SCC. Lesion appears on white light HRE only as a small red blush, much better appreciated with NBI (corresponds to Figure 11.46) (National Cancer Center Hospital East) (Copyright M. Muto).

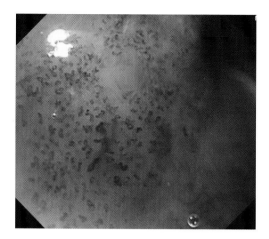

Figure 11.46 Hypopharynx, left pyriform sinus, SCC. Note the sharp demarcation and the abnormal IPCL pattern within the lesion (corresponds to Figure 11.45) (National Cancer Center Hospital East) (Copyright M. Muto).

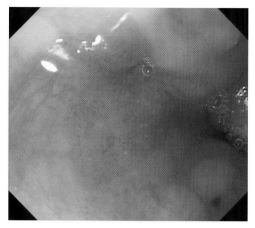

Figure 11.47 Hypopharynx, left pyriform sinus, SCC. The HRE does reveal a demarcation. Examination to detect lesions in the pharynx is best form initially under NBI light (National Cancer Center Hospital East) (Copyright M. Muto).

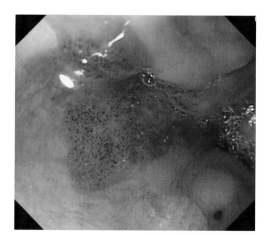

Figure 11.48 Hypopharynx, left pyriform sinus, SCC. The lesion demonstrates a sharp border and dense irregular brown IPCL vessels seen on NBI (corresponds to Figure 11.47) (National Cancer Center Hospital East) (Copyright M. Muto).

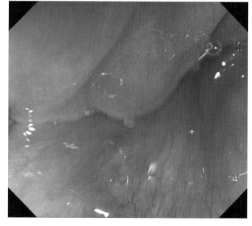

Figure 11.49 Line of discoloration on magnification white light image in right pyriform sinus in this patient with multifocal pharyngeal carcinoma (corresponds to Figure 11.50) (National Cancer Center Hospital East) (Copyright M. Muto).

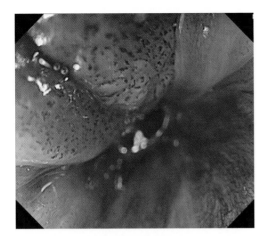

Figure 11.50 NBI magnification view shows irregular IPCL pattern as well as a demarcation line indicative of carcinoma (corresponds to Figure 11.49) (National Cancer Center Hospital East) (Copyright M. Muto).

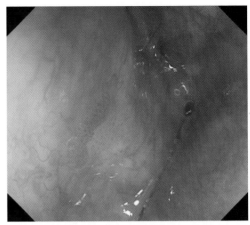

Figure 11.51 Low-magnification white light image shows sharp red line in this patient after chemoradiotherapy for squamous cell carcinoma of the esophagus (corresponds to Figures 11.52 and 11.53) (National Cancer Center Hospital East) (Copyright M. Muto).

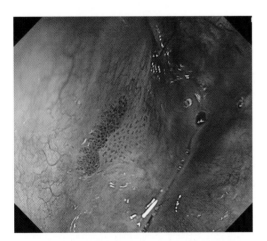

Figure 11.52 NBI view demonstrates a demarcation line with thick irregular brown vessels suspicious for residual carcinoma (National Cancer Center Hospital East) (Copyright M. Muto).

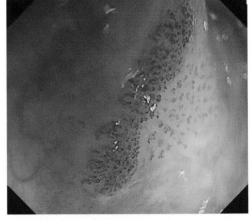

Figure 11.53 Magnified NBI view shows Type 5 IPCL and sharp demarcation in this residual carcinoma post-treatment (National Cancer Center Hospital East) (Copyright M. Muto).

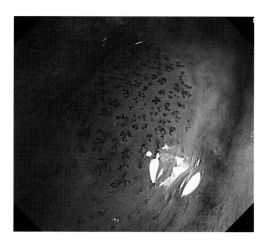

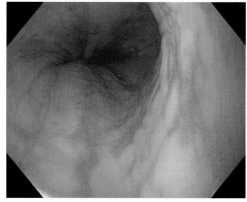

Figure 11.54 Magnified view of this hyperplastic lesion under NBI light to accentuate their irregular IPCL pattern. Note the lack of clear demarcation of the prominent IPCL's (National Cancer Center Hospital East) (Copyright M. Muto).

Figure 11.55 High-resolution white light image demonstrates the furrows of mucosal erosion found in early erosive esophagitis (Mayo Clinic, Jacksonville).

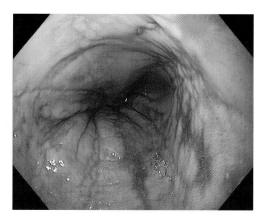

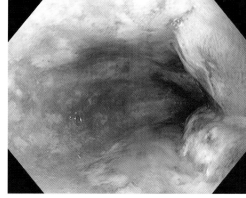

Figure 11.56 The subtle erythematous furrows of early erosive esophagitis are clearly demonstrated with NBI (Mayo Clinic, Jacksonville).

Figure 11.57 Los Angeles Grade 4 gastroesophageal refluxinduced esophagitis (corresponds to Figure 11.58) (University of Utah Health Sciences Center).

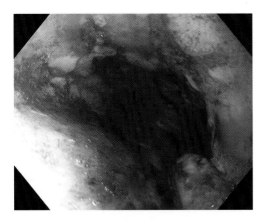

Figure 11.58 NBI low-magnification view of Los Angeles Grade 4 gastro-esophageal reflux-induced esophagitis. As with white light this degree of inflammation precludes meaningful analysis of the surface pattern and vascular pattern to make further diagnoses (corresponds to Figure 11.57) (University of Utah Health Sciences Center).

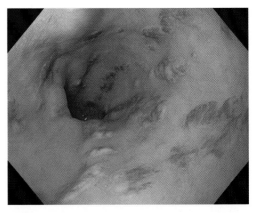

Figure 11.59 High-resolution image demonstrating the white, curd-like exudate of *Candidal* esophagitis. White light veiw is sufficient to make this diagnosis (Mayo Clinic, Jacksonville).

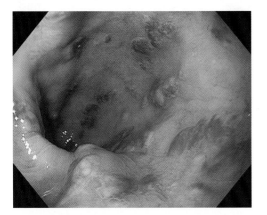

Figure 11.60 *Candida* lesions appear pink on this NBI image given the yellow white light appearance of these lesions. More often, Candida appears white on NBI in stark contrast to the blue gray background (corresponds to Figure 11.59) (Mayo Clinic, Jacksonville).

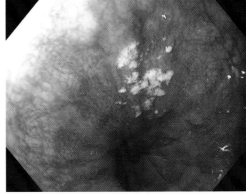

Figure 11.61 Patient with dysmotility of the esophagus found to have these more common white punctate lesions of *Candida* esophagitis (University Medical Center Hamburg Eppendorf).

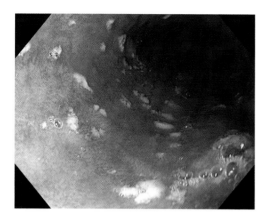

Figure 11.62 Multiple punctate white plaques of *Candida* that stand out under NBI low magnification (NYU School of Medicine).

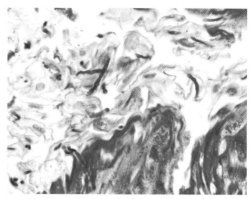

Figure 11.63 *Candida* hyphae and occasional yeast forms in surface and desquamated epithelium (PAS stain) (NYU School of Medicine).

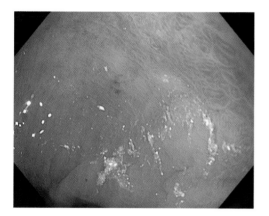

Figure 11.64 Short segment Barrett's esophagus. In this white light view, the villiform Barrett's epithelium is barely discernable proximal to the gastric cardiac epithelium. (University of Utah Health Sciences Center).

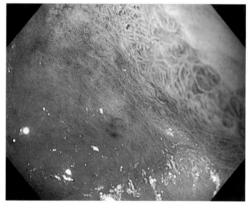

Figure 11.65 NBI non-magnified view of short segment Barrett's esophagus much more clearly delineates the abnormal mucosal pattern than the white light image (University of Utah Health Sciences Center).

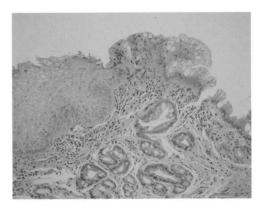

Figure 11.66 Histopathology from a target biopsy of the suspected BE seen on the NBI image shown in Figure 11.65 confirmed the presence of specialized intestinal type metaplasia (University of Utah Health Science Center).

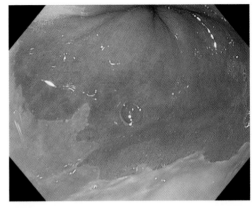

Figure 11.67 High-resolution white light image demonstrating glandular mucosa extending proximally into the tubular esophagus (Mayo Clinic, Jacksonville).

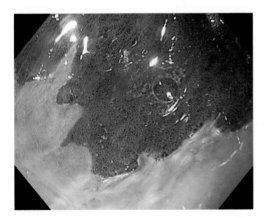

Figure 11.68 Closeup high-resolution NBI that nicely demarcates the squamo-columnar junction and short-segment glandular mucosa with normal mucosal vascular and glandular architecture (corresponds to Figure 11.67) (Mayo Clinic, Jacksonville).

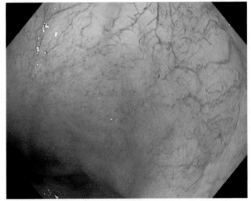

Figure 11.69 This image nicely demonstrates the prominent vascular pattern of short-segment Barrett mucosa compared with the distal cardiac mucosa and adjacent squamous mucosa (corresponds to Figure 11.70) (Mayo Clinic, Jacksonville).

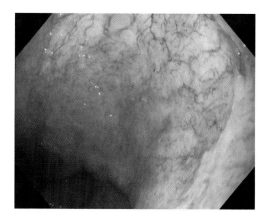

Figure 11.70 NBI highlights the striking vascular pattern of the specialized intestinal metaplasia of Barrett mucosa compared with the distal cardiac mucosa and adjacent squamous mucosa (corresponds to Figure 11.69) (Mayo Clinic, Jacksonville).

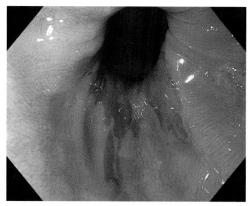

Figure 11.71 NBI image of SSBE. The pink tounges exhibit gyrus/ridge pattern. Type 1 normal IPCLs and Type 2 elongated IPCLs consistent with reflux are seen in the distal squamous mucosa on the left and right sides of the image, respectively (The Johns Hopkins University School of Medicine).

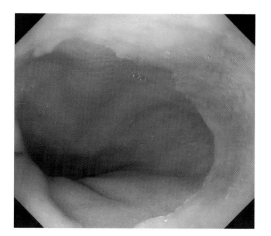

Figure 11.72 SSBE, intestinal metaplasia seen arising just above the top of the gastric folds. On occasion white light images may be useful in identifying the top of these folds to determine whether the pink mucosa in, in fact, BE (National Cancer Center Hospital East) (copyright M. Muto).

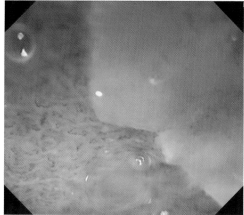

Figure 11.73 SSBE, intestinal metaplasia. Regular vascular pattern and gyrus mucosal pattern readibly discernable on magnification NBI view (National Cancer Center Hospital East) (copyright M. Muto).

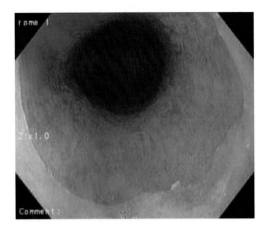

Figure 11.74 Long-segment BE (Catholic University of the Sacred Heart).

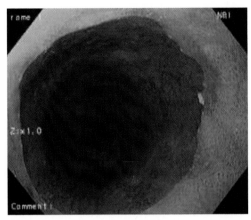

Figure 11.75 Long-segment of BE (Catholic University of the Sacred Heart).

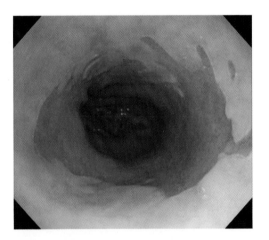

Figure 11.76 Long-segment BE is clearly evident on this low-magnification white light HRE view (University of Amsterdam).

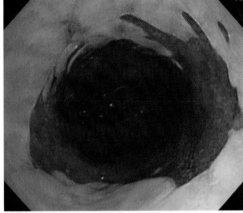

Figure 11.77 NBI in this case provides sharp contrast between squamous and columnar mucosa but is best utilized here to assess mucosal and vessel patterns with magnification over the BE segment (University of Amsterdam).

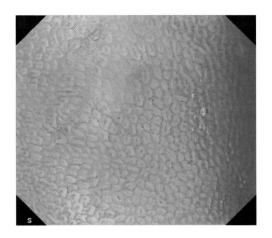

Figure 11.78 White light magnification of regular gyrus pattern of Barrett's epithelium without dysplasia (University of Amsterdam).

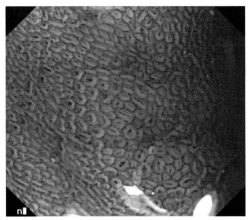

Figure 11.79 Note the smooth and regular surface pattern depicted sharply with magnification NBI consistent with the ridge or gyrus pattern BE (University of Amsterdam).

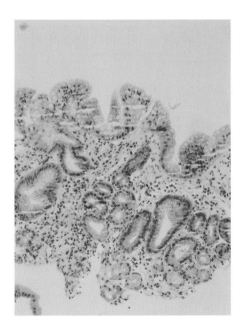

Figure 11.80 Non-dysplastic BE confirmed by histopathology (corresponds to Figures 11.78 and 11.79) (University of Amsterdam).

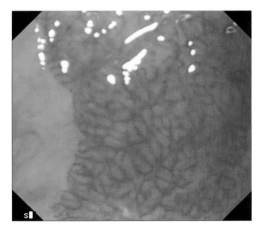

Figure 11.81 White light magnification view can delineate the mucosal pattern in this gyrus type non-dysplastic BE, though NBI is required to properly analyze the vascular pattern (corresponds to Figure 11.82) (University of Amsterdam).

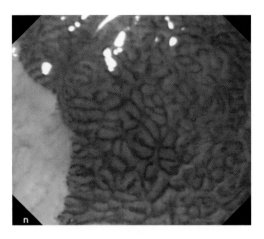

Figure 11.82 This is a variation of the ridge or gyrus pattern of non-dysplastic BE that comprises 80% of all cases. NBI magnified view (University of Amsterdam).

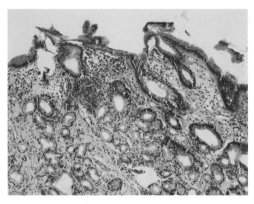

Figure 11.83 Intestinal metaplasia of non-dysplatic BE, low power image. (corresponds to Figures 11.81 and 11.82) (University of Amsterdam).

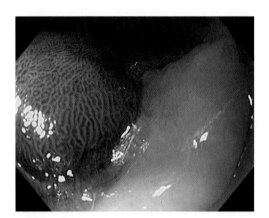

Figure 11.84 Intestinal metaplasia – regular ridge/villous pattern (University of Kansas School of Medicine).

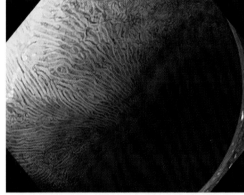

Figure 11.85 Ridge/villous pattern of non-dysplastic BE seen in this magnified NBI view utilizing a cap fitted to the tip of the endoscope touching the surface of the mucosa (University of Kansas School of Medicine).

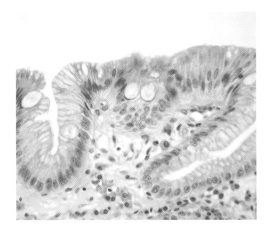

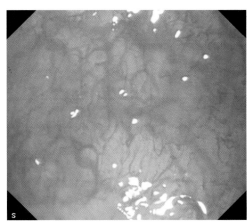

Figure 11.86 Histology corresponding to the ridge/villous pattern in the endoscopic photo (Figure 11.85). Intestinal metaplasia is characterized by bluish goblet cells (University of Kansas School of Medicine).

Figure 11.87 This white light magnified image shows flat mucosa with some hint of prominent vessels but no diagnosis of BE can be made on this basis (University of Amsterdam).

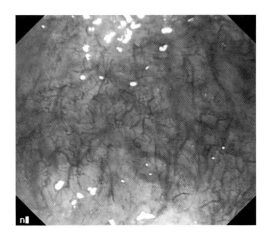

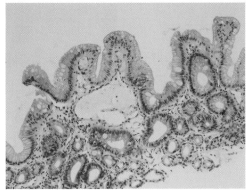

Figure 11.89 Specialized intestinal metaplasia in non-dysplastic BE (corresponds to Figures 11.87 and 11.88) (University of Amsterdam).

Figure 11.88 NBI magnification provides the necessary contrast and definition of vessels to identify the long branching vessels on flat mucosa that comprises 20% of non-dysplastic BE (University of Amsterdam).

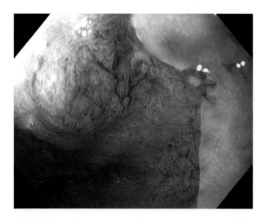

Figure 11.90 Long branching vessel in flat mucosa below the SC junction but above the top of the gastric folds indicative of Barrett's esophagus (NYU School of Medicine).

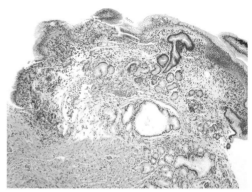

Figure 11.91 Inflamed columnar mucosa near squamo-columnar junction with ectatic blood vessel corresponding to endoscopic NBI image. Adjacent sections show intestinalized epithelium with goblet cells consistent with Barrett's mucosa (NYU School of Medicine).

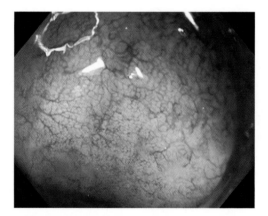

Figure 11.92 Normal vascular pattern of BE without dysplasia (University of Kansas School of Medicine).

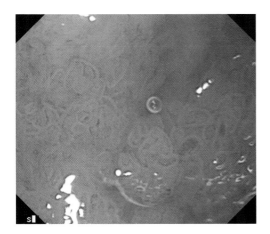

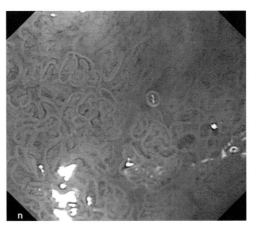

Figure 11.93 Magnification HRE of HGD shows abnormal surface morphology, but it is not possible to assess the vascular pattern on this image (University of Amsterdam).

Figure 11.94 NBI magnification view reveals both the irregular mucosal contour and vascular pattern consistent with the optical diagnosis of HGD (University of Amsterdam).

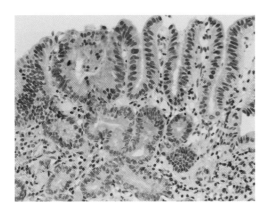

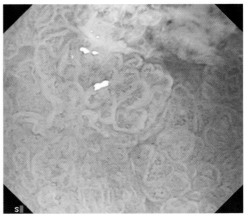

Figure 11.95 HGD is confirmed on histopathology (corresponds to Figures 11.93 and 11.94) (University of Amsterdam).

Figure 11.96 The mucosal surface is raised and irregular in this patient with HGD in BE. White light magnified view (corresponds to Figures 11.97 and 11.98) (University of Amsterdam).

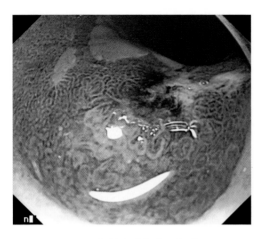

Figure 11.97 NBI highlights the lesions topography. Vascular pattern is best seen under magnification. This view is low magnification (corresponds to Figure 11.96) (University of Amsterdam).

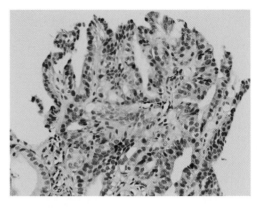

Figure 11.98 HGD suspected on Figures 11.96 and 11.97 is confirmed by histopathology (University of Amsterdam).

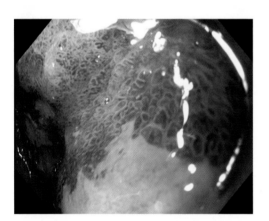

Figure 11.99 Irregular/distorted pattern of mucosa, a key feature of HGD in BE is illustrated in this magnified NBI image (University of Kansas School of Medicine).

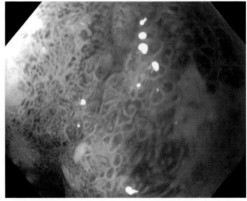

Figure 11.100 The endoscope is pushed closer to the mucosa to gain physical magnification in addition to the digital magnification from this H180 scope. Mucosal irregularities are accentuated (University of Kansas School of Medicine).

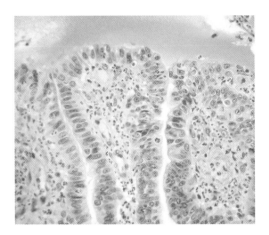

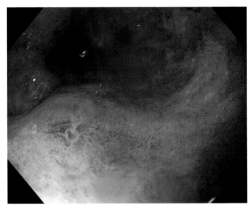

Figure 11.101 HGD at 100 X showing cytologic atypia, loss of nuclear polarity, full thickness stratification of nuclei, and significantly disordered crypt architecture (corresponds to Figures 11.99 and 11.100) (University of Kansas School of Medicine).

Figure 11.102 Note the irregular surface mucosa evident even in low-magnification NBI of this patient with HGD in BE (Medical University of South Carolina).

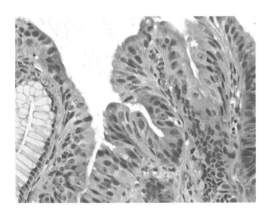

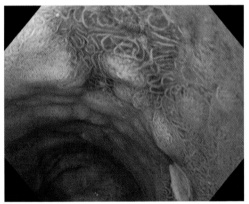

Figure 11.103 The 40× high-power image reveals HGD. There is a mitotic figure in the center of the image, high in the epithelium. There is marked nuclear enlargement with vesicular change and prominent nucleoli (corresponds to Figure 11.102) (Medical University of South Carolina).

Figure 11.104 Low magnification NBI HRE view of long segment BE with focal HGD. Note the depressed and raised areas, wide sulci arranged in a non-parallel irregular pattern (Mayo Clinic, Jacksonville).

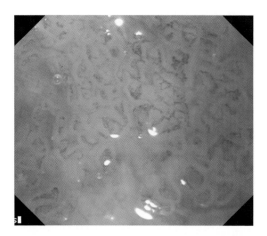

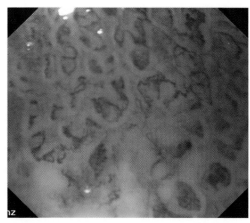

Figure 11.105 White light HRE gives some hint of abnormal vessels but changes seen on this image are very subtle. BE with HGD (University of Amsterdam).

Figure 11.106 Magnification NBI demonstrates abnormally shaped and thickened blood vessels, one key feature of HGD in BE. Note the importance of assessing not only the *pattern* of vessel arrangement, but also the *presence* of abnormal individual vessels (University of Amsterdam).

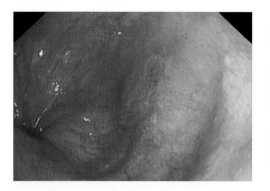

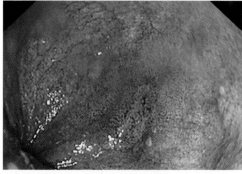

Figure 11.107 This white light image shows what appears may be a simple erosion within BE; the vascular pattern cannot be determined (University of Amsterdam).

Figure 11.108 This HGD in BE displays both a depressed surface and abnormal vessels where the regular mucosal pattern is disrupted (University of Amsterdam).

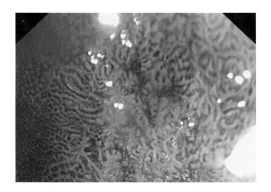

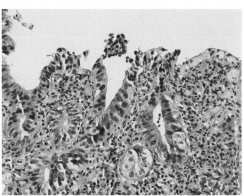

Figure 11.109 Magnified NBI view shows abnormal thick vessels in additional to irregular surface pattern (corresponds to Figures 11.107, 11.108 and 11.110) (University of Amsterdam).

Figure 11.110 Histopathology confirms the suspected HGD (corresponds to Figures 11.107–11.109) (University of Amsterdam).

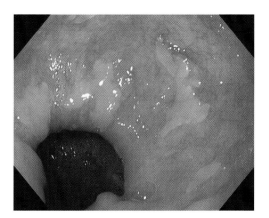

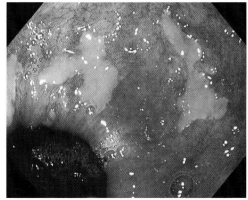

Figure 11.111 BE with abnormal vessels seen in HRE white light without magnification (Mayo Clinic, Jacksonville).

Figure 11.112 NBI improves the ability to detect abnormal vessels in this patient with BE and HGD over white light even without magnification (Mayo Clinic, Jacksonville).

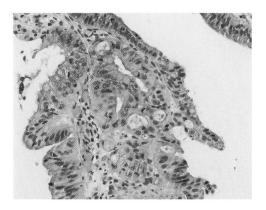

Figure 11.113 Microscopy image demonstrating the special intestinalized metaplasia of Barrett mucosa with focal areas of high-grade dysplasia (corresponds to Figures 11.111–11.112) (Mayo Clinic, Jacksonville).

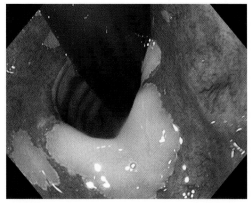

Figure 11.114 This turnaround low-magnification NBI view with prominent vessels to the right of the image within flat mucosa revealed BE indefinite for dysplasia (NYU School of Medicine).

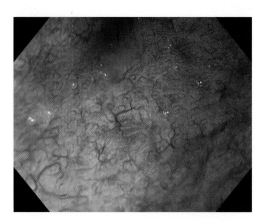

Figure 11.115 Head-on endoscopic magnification NBI view of this area of BE, indefinite for dysplasia (corresponds to Figures 11.114, 11.116, and 11.117) (NYU School of Medicine).

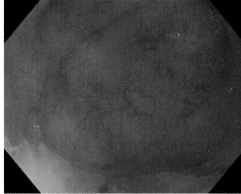

Figure 11.116 White light non-magnified view of this area fails to identify any visible abnormality. The diagnosis would likely have been missed via standard endoscopy (NYU School of Medicine).

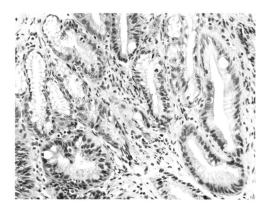

Figure 11.117 Target biopsy within area of Barretts with abnormal vessel as identified with NBI. Note Barrett's mucosa indefinite for dysplasia (corresponds to 11.114–11.116) (NYU School of Medicine).

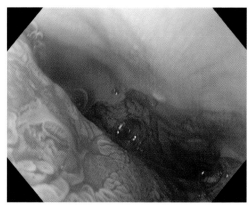

Figure 11.118 Seventy-seven-year-old male patient with a 5 cm Barrett. The Barrett was stained with 1% acetic acid to clear mucous. 1.5× magnification with HRE (University Medical Center Hamburg Eppendorf).

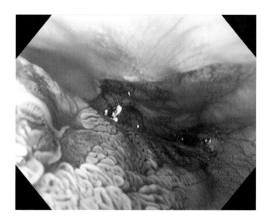

Figure 11.119 NBI, HRE and 1.5 × digital magnification view. On the left is a "blown-up" pattern, more to the right a more "condensed pattern." Histopathology showed low-grade dysplasia in this lesion with abnormal mucosal pattern (corresponds to 11.118) (University Medical Center Hamburg Eppendorf).

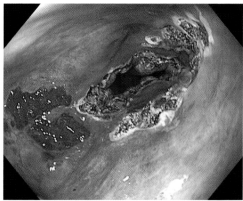

Figure 11.120 Residual BE after ablation being treated with argon plasma coagulation. Untreated patches remain visible to the left of this photo (corresponds to Figure 11.121) (Mayo Clinic, Jacksonville).

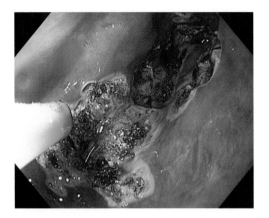

Figure 11.121 APC to the remaining areas of residual BE which are easy to detect using NBI under low magnification (corresponds to Figure 11.120) (Mayo Clinic, Jacksonville).

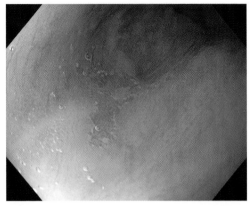

Figure 11.122 White light HRE view of a patient with residual BE following ablation (Mayo Clinic, Jacksonville).

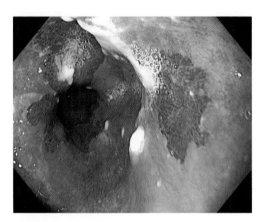

Figure 11.123 NBI much more clearly delineates the residual BE following ablation for targeted biopsy or further treatment (corresponds to Figure 11.122) (Mayo Clinic, Jacksonville).

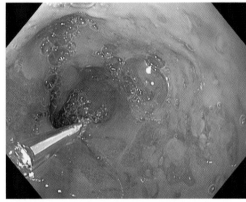

Figure 11.124 White light HRE image of PDT for Barrett's esophagus ablation (corresponds to Figure 11.125) (Mayo Clinic, Jacksonville).

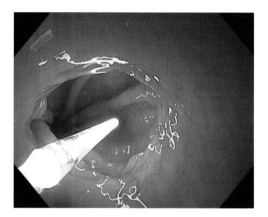

Figure 11.125 While NBI is very useful following PDT for assessment of residual BE, during treatment it has limited added value over white light once the extent and location of the target has been measured (corresponds to Figure 11.124) (Mayo Clinic, Jacksonville).

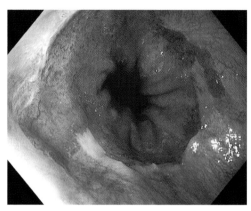

Figure 11.126 NBI low magnification is used to identify this short segment of Barrett's epithelium (corresponds to Figures 11.127–11.131) (Dartmouth Hitchcock Medical Center).

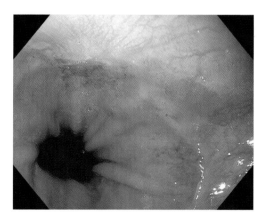

Figure 11.127 This same segment is shown in white light HRE close up prior to Barrx radio frequency ablation of the BE (Dartmouth Hitchcock Medical Center).

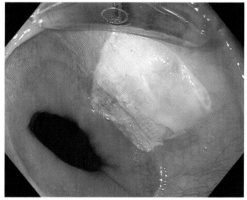

Figure 11.128 HRE image of HALO 90 radio frequency ablation after first application with device attached to the tip of the scope positioned at 12 o'clock and seen in the top center of this photo (Dartmouth Hitchcock Medical Center).

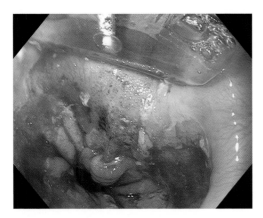

Figure 11.129 Chamois-colored area demonstrating change after second RF application at 12 o'clock position, white light HRE low-magnification view (Dartmouth Hitchcock Medical Center).

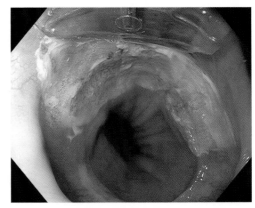

Figure 11.130 The ablation continues in a counter-clockwise direction (Dartmouth Hitchcock Medical Center).

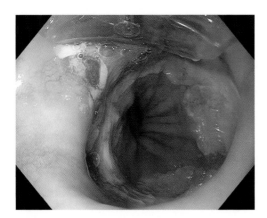

Figure 11.131 White light HRE image of the entire segment of SSIM immediately following RF ablation (corresponds to Figures 11.126–11.130) (Dartmouth Hitchcock Medical Center).

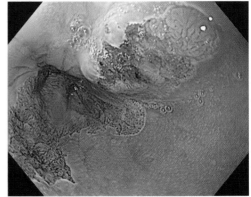

Figure 11.132 This area of focal irregular raised and erythroplastic mucosa in BE is shown here in NBI low magnification view (corresponds to Figure 11.133) (Edward Herriot Hospital).

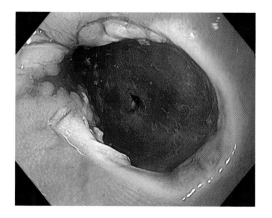

Figure 11.133 White light HRE view of this area following capEMR of what was found to be a superficial adenocarcinoma (corresponds to Figure 11.132) (Edouard Herriot Hospital).

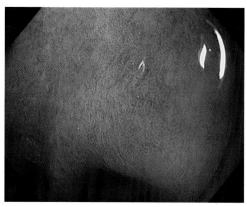

Figure 11.134 Tight circular pattern of normal cardia well delineated on magnification NBI image (University of Kansas School of Medicine).

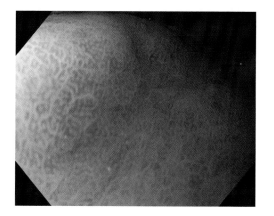

Figure 11.135 NBI close up 1.5× magnified view of cardia mucosa just below SC junction reveals some thick sulci but round cardia-type mucosal pattern (NYU School of Medicine).

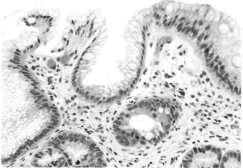

Figure 11.136 Histopathology confirms the presence of cardiac mucosa with scant inflammation and intestinal metaplasia negative for dysplasia (corresponds to Figure 11.135) (NYU School of Medicine).

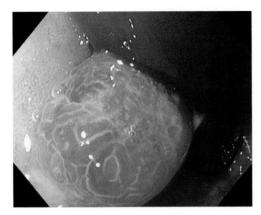

Figure 11.137 View in retroversion of mucosal adenocarcinoma in Barretts on white light (University Medical Center Hamburg Eppendorf).

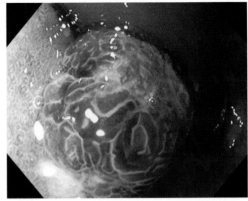

Figure 11.138 Mucosal cancer of the cardia arising from BE with grossly irregular gyrus mucosal pattern on NBI view (corresponds to Figure 11.137) (University Medical Center Hamburg Eppendorf).

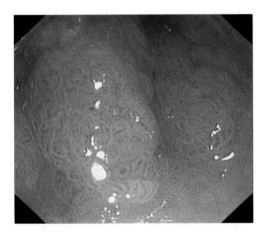

Figure 11.139 White light magnified HRE outlines the abnormal mucosal topography of this adenocarcinoma of the cardia (University of Amsterdam).

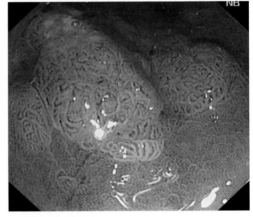

Figure 11.140 NBI magnification view both accentuates the abnormal topography apparent under white light (Figure 11.139) and reveals the irregular, thickened vessels arranged in an abnormal pattern (University of Amsterdam).

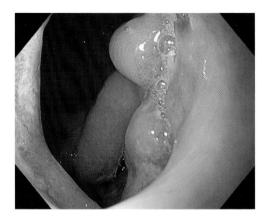

Figure 11.141 Nodular adenocarcinoma at the GEJ – esophageal view (Mayo Clinic, Jacksonville).

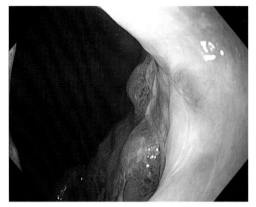

Figure 11.142 NBI of nodular GEJ carcinoma from distal esophagus (Mayo Clinic, Jacksonville).

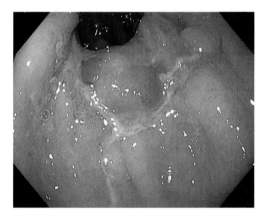

Figure 11.143 Nodular GEJ carcinoma, retroflexed view from the cardia (corresponds to Figures 11.141–11.146) (Mayo Clinic, Jacksonville).

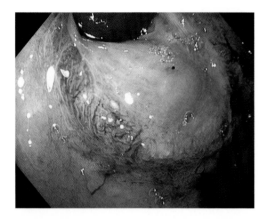

Figure 11.144 NBI of GEJ nodular carcinoma, retroflexed view from the cardia shows
much greater definition of the lesion, its vessels, and its margins (corresponds to Figures
11.141–11.146) (Mayo Clinic, Jacksonville).

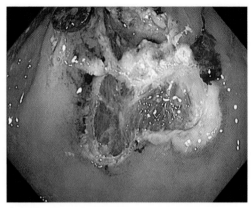

Figure 11.145 HRE image after band-
EMR, view from the cardia (Mayo Clinic,
Jacksonville).

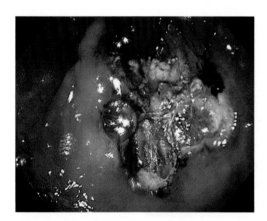

Figure 11.146 NBI of nodular carcinoma after EMR. NBI is particularly useful in examining for any residual tumor or
polyp following resection (Mayo Clinic,
Jacksonville).

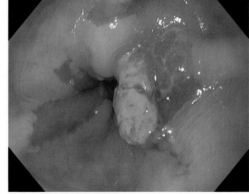

Figure 11.147 White raised esophageal
adenocarcinoma arising in BE here seen in
white light on low magnification (corresponds
to Figure 11.148) (Medical University of South
Carolina).

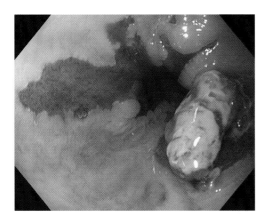

Figure 11.148 NBI low-magnification view of this lesion is well demarcated, but does not add much over this clearly discernable lesion (corresponds to Figure 11.147) (Medical University of South Carolina).

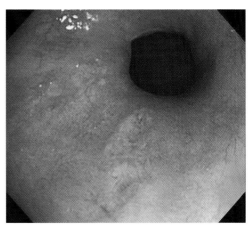

Figure 11.149 White light HRE image of this esophageal adenocarcinoma detects an abnormality but the appearance is not well distinguished from a benign erosion in this view (University of Amsterdam).

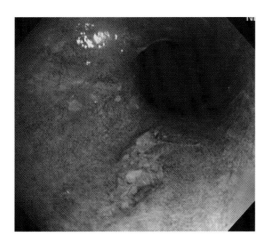

Figure 11.150 NBI of this adenocarcinoma. The lesion demonstrates depressed irregular mucosa and irregular vessel pattern (corresponds to Figure 11.149) (University of Amsterdam).

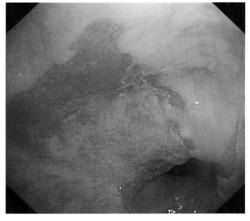

Figure 11.151 This white light HRE image of an adenocarcinoma clearly shows BE with some apparent squamous reepithelialization. The abnormal morphology is much better appreciated with NBI (corresponds to Figure 11.152) (University of Amsterdam).

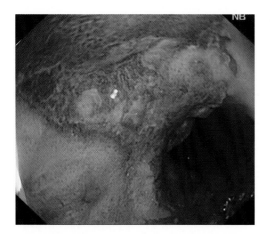

Figure 11.152 This adenocarcinoma arising out of BE displays marked abnormal morphology and vascular pattern even on low magnification view (corresponds to Figure 11.151) (University of Amsterdam).

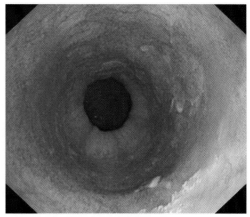

Figure 11.153 An early esophageal adenocarcinoma discernable in this white light low-magnification image as a flat discoloration and slightly irregular surface at 3 o'clock (University of Amsterdam).

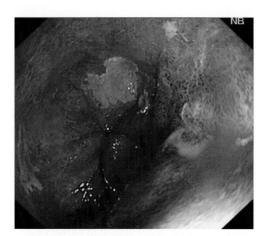

Figure 11.154 NBI more clearly defines the lesion by highlighting the mucosal surface change and increased vessel density (corresponds to Figures 11.153 and 11.155) (University of Amsterdam).

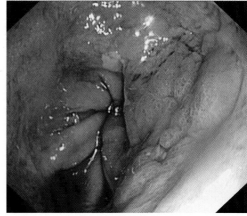

Figure 11.155 Chromoendoscopy reveals pit pattern and more clearly defines the neoplastic lesion (University of Amsterdam).

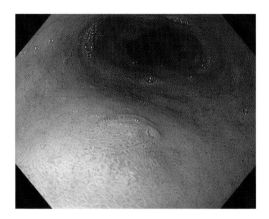

Figure 11.156 A raised irregular superficial lesion is seen in this esophagus under white light low magnification (Edouard Herriot Hospital).

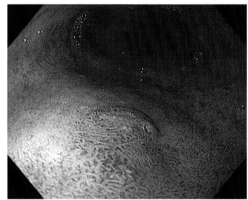

Figure 11.157 NBI low-magnification image of this nodular superficial carcinoma (IIa lesion) arising in BE. Improved delineation of margins and characterization of surface morphology over white light is demonstrated (Edouard Herriot Hospital).

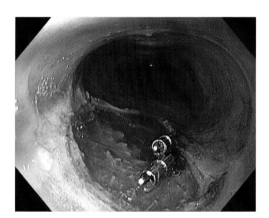

Figure 11.158 White light image of lesion immediately following EMR. Clips have been applied to control bleeding (corresponds to Figures 11.156–11.160) (Edouard Herriot Hospital).

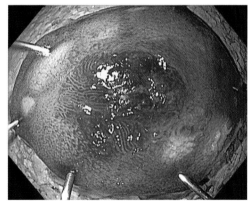

Figure 11.159 Magnified white light examination of the resection specimen (Edouard Herriot Hospital).

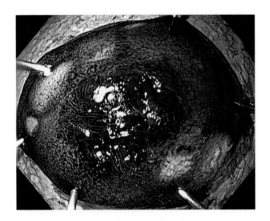

Figure 11.160 NBI of completely resected lesion with margins (corresponds to Figures 11.156–11.159) (Edouard Herriot Hospital).

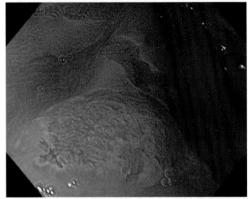

Figure 11.161 White light low-magnification view of nodular isolated superficial carcinoma arising in BE (Edouard Herriot Hospital).

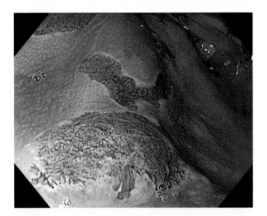

Figure 11.162 NBI low-magnification image provides more precise characterization. The surface appears irregular and contrasts with the normal BE tongue at the top of the photo (loss of the regular villous or gyrus pattern of non-dysplastic BE) (corresponds to Figures 11.161–11.164) (Edouard Herriot Hospital).

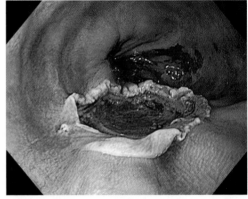

Figure 11.163 NBI is used to assess for any residual tissue following successful EMR of this lesion (Edouard Herriot Hospital).

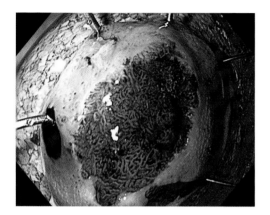

Figure 11.164 NBI examination of the fully resected superficial carcinoma (corresponds to Figures 11.161–11.163) (Edouard Herriot Hospital).

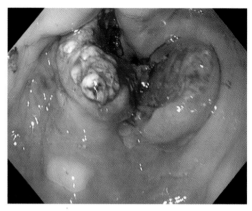

Figure 11.165 Special contrast is not needed to diagnose this near-obstructing esophageal carcinoma seen here in low-magnification white light (Mayo Clinic, Jacksonville).

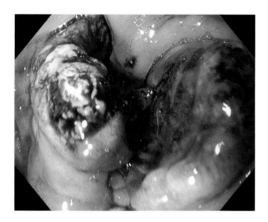

Figure 11.166 Obstructing esophageal adeno-carcinoma, NBI view with markedly abnormal vessels and macroscopic appearance consistent with invasive malignant disease (corresponds to Figure 11.165) (Mayo Clinic, Jacksonville).

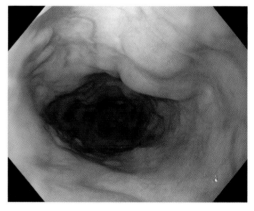

Figure 11.167 White light HRE low-magnification image of a patient with esophageal varices. Note the one prominent column in the one o'clock position (corresponds to Figure 11.168) (Mayo Clinic, Jacksonville).

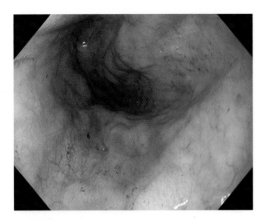

Figure 11.168 Esophageal varices, seen on NBI light without obvious advantage over white light view (corresponds to Figure 11.167) (Mayo Clinic, Jacksonville).

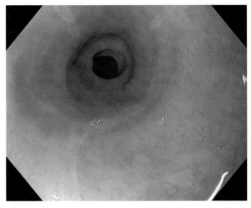

Figure 11.169 Normal magnification white light provides a good assessment of this smooth benign esophageal stricture (Mayo Clinic, Jacksonville).

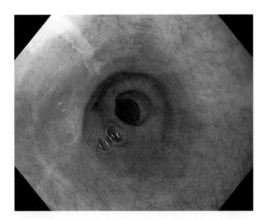

Figure 11.170 Esophageal stricture benign, NBI low-magnification view. The surface structure and vascular pattern appears normal (corresponds to Figure 11.169) (Mayo Clinic, Jacksonville).

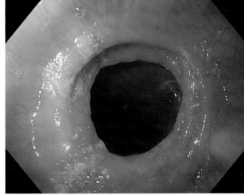

Figure 11.171 Rings in distal esophagus in patients with confirmed eosinophilic esophagitis, white light non-magnified view (NYU School of Medicine).

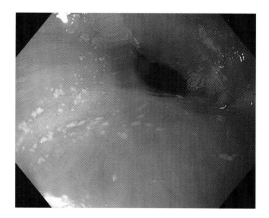

Figure 11.172 Multiple tiny white plaques suggesting Candidiasis actually represent eosinophilic esophageal microabscesses. White light non-magnified view (NYU School of Medicine).

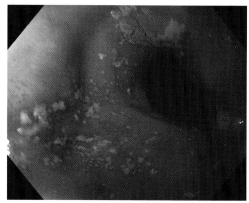

Figure 11.173 Eosinophilic esophagitis, narrow band non-magnified view (NYU School of Medicine).

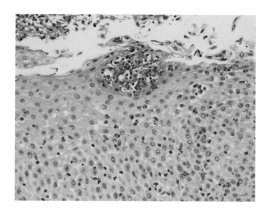

Figure 11.174 Eosinophilic esophagitis. Numerous eosinophils are distributed throughout the epithelium, with aggregates forming microabscesses at the surface (corresponds to Figures 11.172 and 11.173) (NYU School of Medicine).

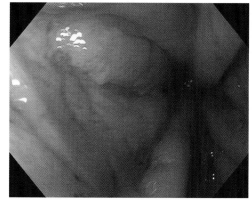

Figure 11.175 Pediatric patient with a clinical presentation of dysphagia found to have eosinophilic esophagitis. NBI low-magnification view (The Johns Hopkins University School of Medicine).

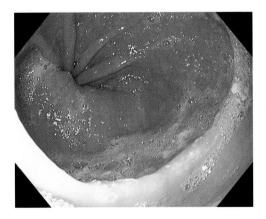

Figure 11.176 NBI non-magnified view of Schatski ring (NYU School of Medicine).

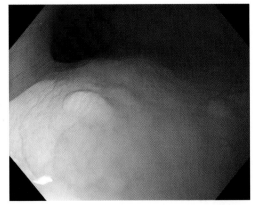

Figure 11.177 Squamous papilloma of the esophagus viewed with white light, low magnification (University of Utah Health Sciences Center).

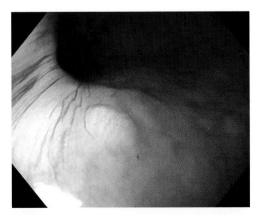

Figure 11.178 Squamous papilloma of the esophagus viewed with NBI light. Note the confluent color of the mucosal and the papilloma (University of Utah Health Sciences Center).

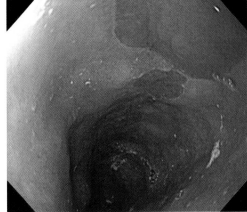

Figure 11.179 White light low-magnification endoscopy reveals a gastric inlet patch upon slow withdrawal of the endoscope from the esophagus (corresponds to Figure 11.180) (Mount Sinai School of Medicine).

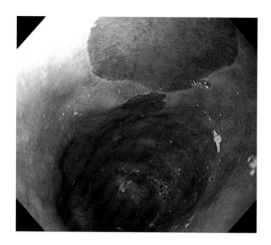

Figure 11.180 Gastric inlet patch (NBI image). While the preceding white light image (Figure 11.179) shows the same lesion, the stark contrast makes this finding hard to miss (Mount Sinai School of Medicine).

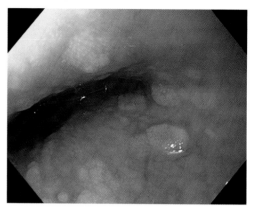

Figure 11.181 White light non-magnifying image of esophageal glycogen deposits (NYU School of Medicine).

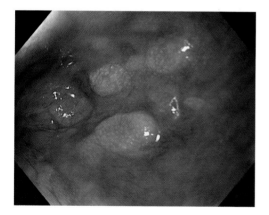

Figure 11.182 NBI view of esophageal glycogen deposits (NYU School of Medicine).

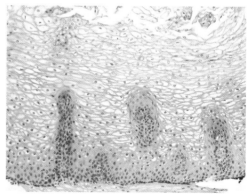

Figure 11.183 The supra-basal squamous cells are distended with barely visible eosinophilic cytoplasm due to glycogen accumulation (corresponds to Figures 11.181 and 11.182) (NYU School of Medicine).

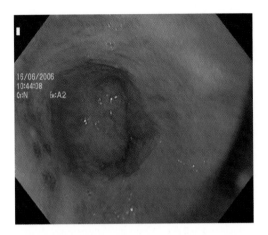

Figure 11.184 Esophageal angiodysplasia in Rendu-Osler-Weber syndrome seen on white light HRE view (Hospital Sao Marcos).

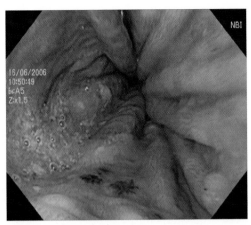

Figure 11.185 NBI low-magnification view of esophageal angiodysplasia in Rendu-Osler-Weber syndrome (Hospital Sao Marcos).

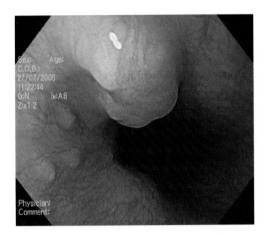

Figure 11.186 Esophageal leiomyoma seen here with HRE white light without magnification (Hospital Sao Marcos).

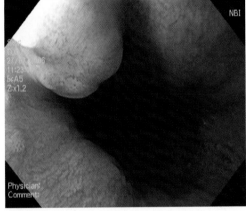

Figure 11.187 Low-magnification NBI view of this esophageal leiomyoma (Hospital Sao Marcos).

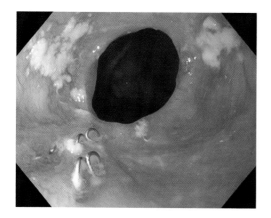

Figure 11.188 Esophageal-gastric anastamosis with staples and yeast, HRE white light low-magnification view (Mayo Clinic, Jacksonville).

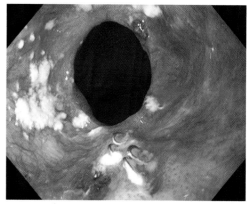

Figure 11.189 NBI image here easily detects abnormalities on the surface in low magnification in this narrow lumen where there is sufficient light for its contrast to be effective in scanning the mucosa for lesions (Mayo Clinic, Jacksonville).

ABBREVIATIONS USED

APC:	argon plasma coagulation
EMR:	endoscopic mucosal resection
GERD:	gastro-esophageal reflux disease
HRE:	high-resolution endoscopy
IPCLs:	intra-epithelial papillary capillary loops
NBI:	narrow band imaging
PDT:	photodynamic therapy
PAS:	periodic acid schiff
RF:	adio frequency
SCC:	squamous cell carcinoma
SSBE:	short segment Barrett's esophagus
GEJ:	gastro-esophageal junction

Stomach atlas

12

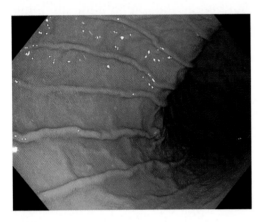

Figure 12.1 HRE white light image of the folds of the gastric body, greater curvature (NYU School of Medicine).

Figure 12.2 NBI image of the same view is far too dark to reveal mucosal detail; the gastric lumen is too wide to utilize NBI as screen for lesion detection in contrast to narrower lumen organs such as the esophagus or colon (NYU School of Medicine).

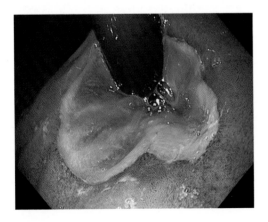

Figure 12.3 Normal cardia turnaround NBI low-magnification image (NYU School of Medicine).

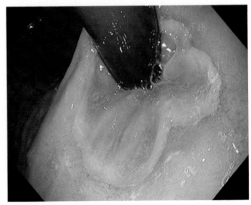

Figure 12.4 Normal cardia seen in retroflex view, white light (NYU School of Medicine).

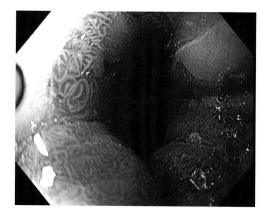

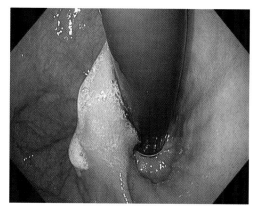

Figure 12.5 NBI image of carditis. Note the thickened round mucosal pattern of inflamed cardia mucosa (Institut Arnault Tzanck).

Figure 12.6 Retroflex white light low-magnification view of cardia with pathology confirmed chronic inflammation (NYU School of Medicine).

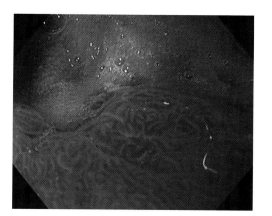

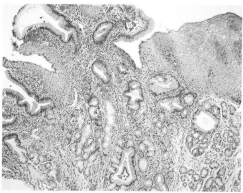

Figure 12.7 NBI 1.5× magnified view in turn-around of chronic inflammation of cardia mucosa (NYU School of Medicine).

Figure 12.8 Reflux carditis. There is intense acute and chronic inflammation of the cardiac mucosa at the squamo-columnar junction (corresponds to Figures 12.6 and 12.7) (NYU School of Medicine).

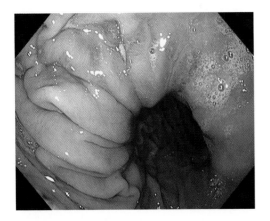

Figure 12.9 Cameron lesions, HRE white light low-magnification view (Mayo Clinic, Jacksonville).

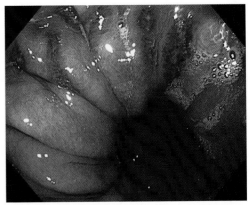

Figure 12.10 Cameron lesions, NBI view (Mayo Clinic, Jacksonville).

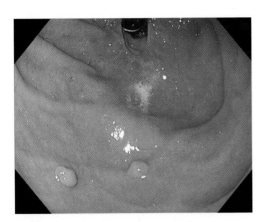

Figure 12.11 HRE white light low-magnification image of normal fundus with two small fundic gland polyps and hiatal hernia seen in turnaround view (Mayo Clinic, Jacksonville).

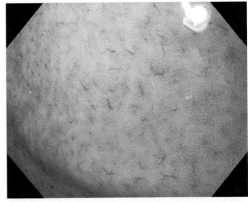

Figure 12.12 This magnification NBI image of the fundic mucosa reveals normal vascular pattern and surface pattern. Corresponding histopathology confirmed normal mucosa (NYU School of Medicine).

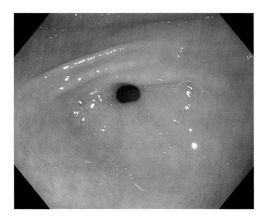

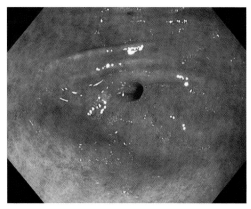

Figure 12.13 White light view of a normal gastric antrum (University of Utah Health Sciences Center).

Figure 12.14 Normal gastric antrum, NBI low-magnification view (University of Utah Health Sciences Center).

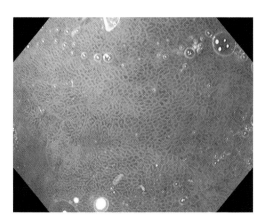

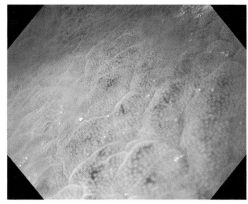

Figure 12.15 Normal antrum magnification NBI image shows regular pattern with narrow sulci (NYU School of Medicine).

Figure 12.16 Magnified NBI view in the antral body transition of active *Helicobacter pylori* infection. Note bumpy surface topography, widened pits and focal increased vascular markings (vessels in dark) (corresponds to Figure 12.17) (NYU School of Medicine).

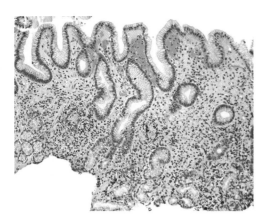

Figure 12.17 *Helicobacter*-associated active chronic antral gastritis (corresponds to Figure 12.16) (NYU School of Medicine).

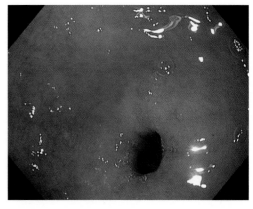

Figure 12.18 White light HRE low-magnification image of antrum in a patient with dyspepsia and NSAID medication use. No erosions or ulcerations noted (NYU School of Medicine).

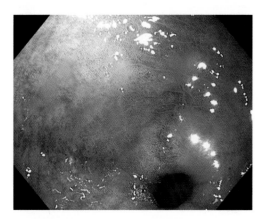

Figure 12.19 Patchy darkened areas in the antrum of this patient who had been taking NSAID medications. No ulcers present. NBI accentuates unevenness and furrows in the mucosa (NYU School of Medicine).

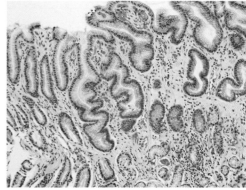

Figure 12.20 Reactive gastropathy. The gastric mucosa is hyperplastic with tortuous glands, diminished mucin in the foveolar epithelium and muscularization of the lamina propria (corresponds to Figures 12.18 and 12.19) (NYU School of Medicine).

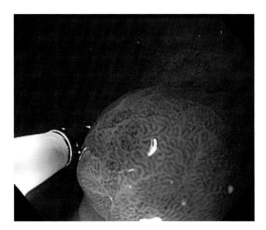

Figure 12.21 Raised area of antral mucosa without erosion in this patient taking non-steroidal anti-inflammatory medications (NYU School of Medicine).

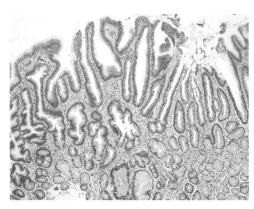

Figure 12.22 Histopathology of this lesion shows reactive gastropathy. Elongated, tortuous antral glands are lined by epithelium with mild reactive atypia. Consistent with chemical gastritis (NYU School of Medicine).

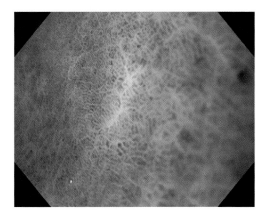

Figure 12.23 Antral scar representing healed erosion, *Helicobacter pylori* negative, NBI 1.5× magnification view (NYU School of Medicine).

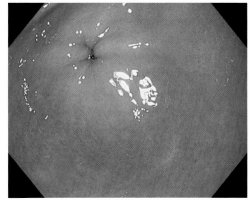

Figure 12.24 Antrum in patient with healed erosion not apparent in white light low-magnification view (NYU School of Medicine).

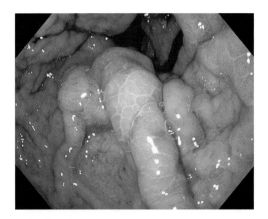

Figure 12.25 Fundic varices, HRE view (Mayo Clinic, Jacksonville).

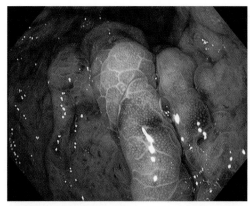

Figure 12.26 Fundic varices, NBI view (Mayo Clinic, Jacksonville).

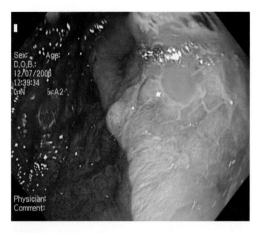

Figure 12.27 Severe portal hypertension gastropathy, white light low-magnification view (Hospital Sao Marcos).

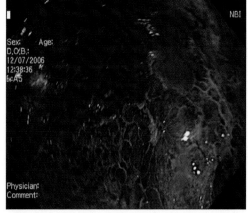

Figure 12.28 Severe portal hypertension gastropathy, NBI low-magnification view demonstrating leopard skin appearance. In this case due to the darker images in the stomach related to the larger lumen, white light better illustrates the finding (Hospital Sao Marcos).

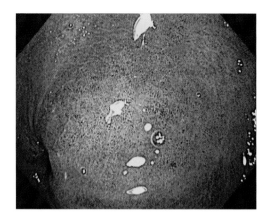

Figure 12.29 Subeptihelial hemorrhages in portal hypertensive gastropathy, NBI view low magnification (Institut Arnault Tzanck).

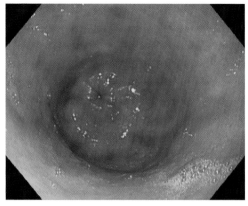

Figure 12.30 White light HRE low-magnification view of portal hypertensive gastropathy, GAVE pattern (Institut Arnault Tzanck).

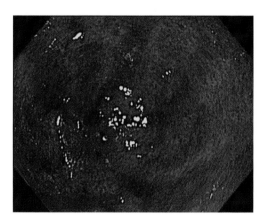

Figure 12.31 Portal hypertensive gastropathy with GAVE pattern, NBI low-magnification view (corresponds to Figure 12.30) (Institut Arnault Tzanck).

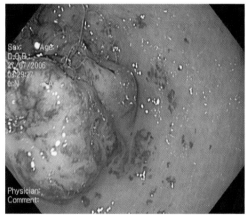

Figure 12.32 GAVE HRE low-magnification view (corresponds to Figure 12.33) (Hospital Sao Marcos).

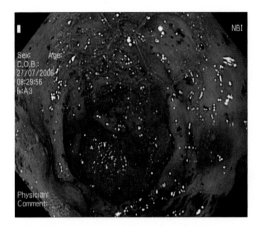

Figure 12.33 GAVE NBI HRE low-magnification view (corresponds to Figure 12.32) (Hospital Sao Marcos).

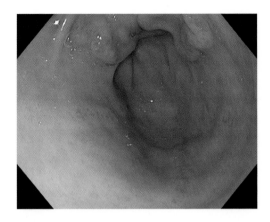

Figure 12.34 Subtle changes of GAVE on white light HRE, may become more evident with NBI (Lenox Hill Hospital).

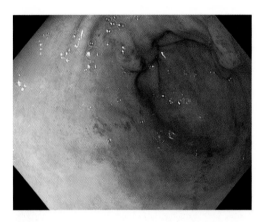

Figure 12.35 Subtle changes of GAVE more evident on NBI (corresponds to Figure 12.34) (Lenox Hill Hospital).

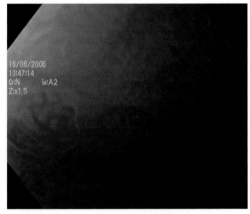

Figure 12.36 Gastric angiodysplasia in Rendu–Osler–Weber syndrome seen well in white light magnification HRE view (corresponds to Figure 12.37) (Hospital Sao Marcos).

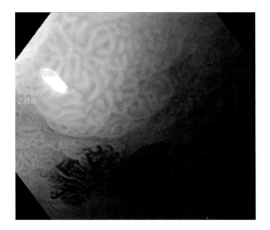

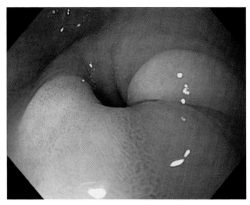

Figure 12.37 NBI magnified view of the same lesion, now black in appearance instead of red (corresponds to Figure 12.36) (Hospital Sao Marcos).

Figure 12.38 Pyloric erosion faintly visible on white light HRE (Erasmus University Hospital).

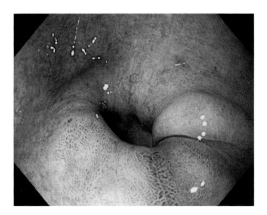

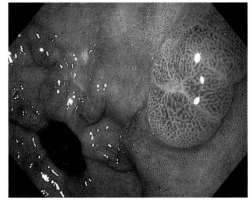

Figure 12.39 Pyloric erosion more easily seen on NBI low magnification view than on white light (corresponds to Figure 12.38) (Erasmus University Hospital).

Figure 12.40 Focal antral erosion in patient with portal hypertension taking non-steroidal anti-inflammatory medications, NBI 1.5× magnification (NYU School of Medicine).

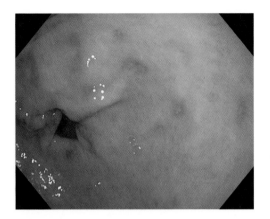

Figure 12.41 Multiple antral gastric erosions related to NSAIDs, HRE white light non-magnified view (Mayo Clinic, Jacksonville).

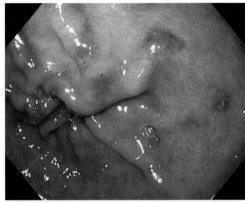

Figure 12.42 Multiple NSAID-associated antral gastric erosions, NBI low-maginification view (Mayo Clinic, Jacksonville).

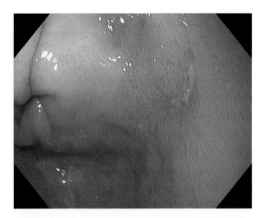

Figure 12.43 Benign appearing chronic gastric ulcer, white light (NYU School of Medicine).

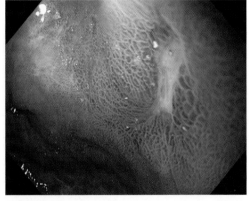

Figure 12.44 Chronic benign appearing gastric ulcer, NBI non-magnified view. Pathology demonstrated foveolar hyperplasia, active chronic gastritis and focal intestinal metaplasia (NYU School of Medicine).

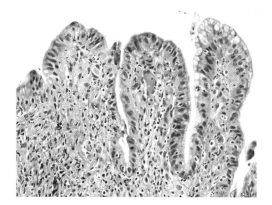

Figure 12.45 Acutely inflamed mucosa of benign gastric ulcer with marked reactive epithelial atypia is present at the ulcer edge (corresponds to Figures 12.43 and 12.44) (NYU School of Medicine).

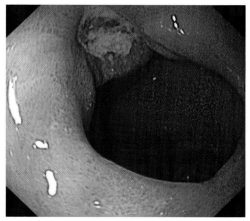

Figure 12.46 Non-magnified white light view of benign appearing gastric ulcer with smooth regular borders (Institut Arnault Tzanck).

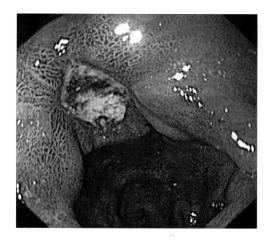

Figure 12.47 Well demarcated NBI image of benign solitary gastric ulcer, non-magnified view. The flat nature of the pigmented spot is clearly seen (corresponds to Figure 12.46) (Institut Arnault Tzanck).

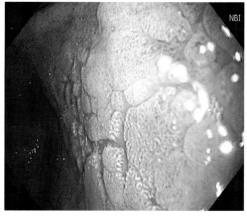

Figure 12.48 HRE low-magnification view of gastric intestinal metaplasia (Hospital Sao Marcos).

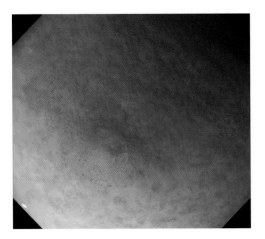

Figure 12.49 Chronic inflammation. This raised red lesion might raise suspicions for early cancer on first glance (National Cancer Center Hospital East) (copyright M. Muto).

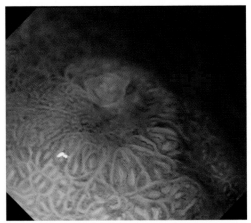

Figure 12.50 Magnification NBI image shows it to be an erosion due to chronic inflammation; notice the regular surrounding mucosal pattern and while the central area loses this pattern, there are no abnormal microvessels (National Cancer Center Hospital East) (copyright M. Muto).

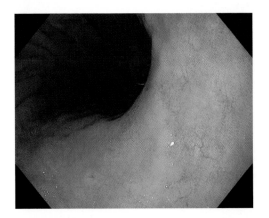

Figure 12.51 Low-grade dysplasia under white light low-magnification view. The lesion is slightly depressed with a reddened color (Lenox Hill Hospital).

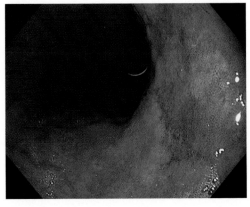

Figure 12.52 NBI close-up image is more valuable than white light view in assessing for low grade dysplasia. (Lenox Hill Hospital).

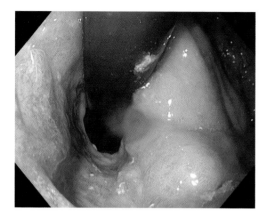

Figure 12.53 Hiatal hernia with intramucosal carcinoma in the cardia, HRE white
light low-magnification image (Mayo Clinic,
Jacksonville).

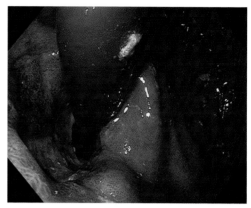

Figure 12.54 NBI low-magnification view
more clearly delineates the abnormal area.
Magnification is required to assess the microvascular pattern (Mayo Clinic, Jacksonville).

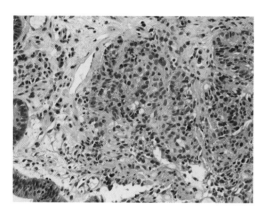

Figure 12.55 Histologic section from
cardia demonstrating high-grade dysplasia
suspicious for intramucosal carcinoma (corresponds to Figures 12.53 and 12.54) (Mayo
Clinic, Jacksonville).

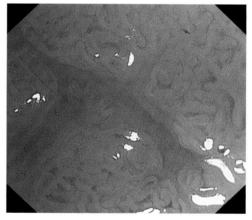

Figure 12.56 Delineation of gastric cancer,
demarcation line seen well with magnification
white light. Microvessels better assessed with
NBI (corresponds to Figure 12.57) (University
of Amsterdam).

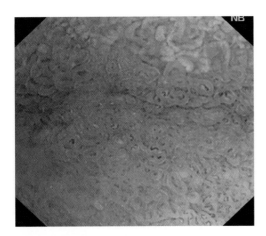

Figure 12.57 Delineation of early gastric cancer with sharp demarcation line at loss of mucosal pattern, NBI magnification view (corresponds to Figure 12.56) (University of Amsterdam).

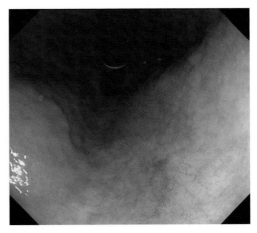

Figure 12.58 This small discoloration in the upper stomach could reflect a benign erosion, a telangiectasia or an early neoplasm (National Cancer Center Hospital East) (copyright M. Muto).

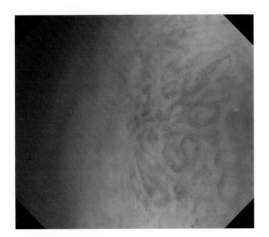

Figure 12.59 Magnification demonstrates no erosion to mucosal surface which has a regular pattern (National Cancer Center Hospital East) (copyright M. Muto).

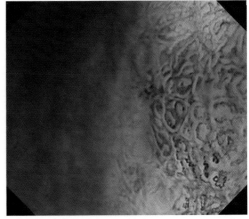

Figure 12.60 This is a gastric telangiectasia. While there are a few abnormal microvessels there is no demarcation line, and indication that this is a non-neoplastic lesion (corresponds to Figures 12.58 and 12.59) (National Cancer Center Hospital East) (copyright M. Muto).

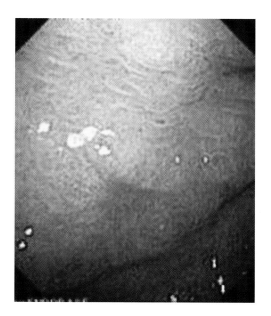

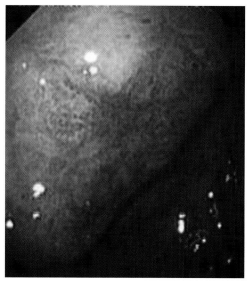

Figure 12.61 Endoscopic view of a superficial IIa–IIc lesion in the gastric antrum (Catholic University of the Sacred Heart).

Figure 12.62 NBI view of a superficial IIa–IIc lesion in the gastric antrum. Vascular pattern more discernable in depressed portion (Catholic University of the Sacred Heart).

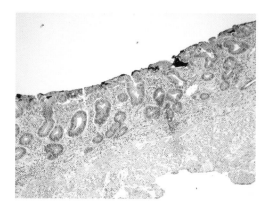

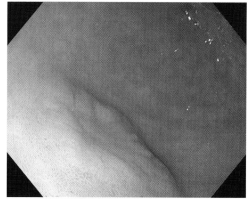

Figure 12.63 EMR specimen showing moderately differentiated adenocarcinoma limited to the epithelial layer (corresponds to Figures 12.61 and 12.62) (Catholic University of the Sacred Heart).

Figure 12.64 Superficial gastric carcinoma on the greater curvature IIa–IIc mixed raised and depressed lesion, seen in white light low-maginification view (corresponds to Figures 12.65–12.67) (Edouard Herriot Hospital).

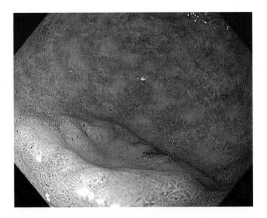

Figure 12.65 Superficial gastric carcinoma IIa–IIc on the greater curvature: the lesion appears whitish and is better delineated than with white light (Edouard Herriot Hospital).

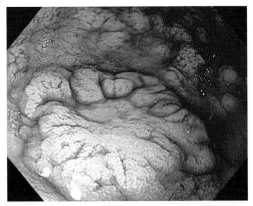

Figure 12.66 Superficial gastric carcinoma IIa–IIc on the greater curvature: the lesion is better delineated than with NBI, especially in terms of the surface assessment of the raised portion. Indigo>NBI>white light (Edouard Herriot Hospital).

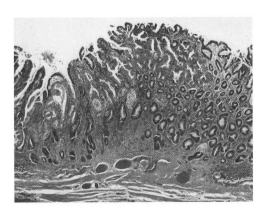

Figure 12.67 Early gastric cancer, in this case confined to the mucosa (corresponds to Figures 12.64–12.66) (Edouard Herriot Hospital).

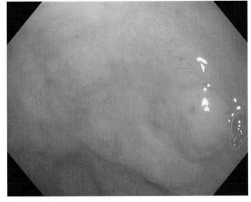

Figure 12.68 This gastric superficial carcinoma IIa–IIc appears on white light view as discoloration and slightly irregular surface (corresponds to Figures 12.69 and 12.70) (Edouard Herriot Hospital).

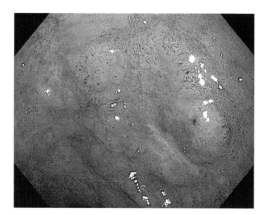

Figure 12.69 Superficial gastric carcinoma IIa–IIc: the lesion appears whitish and is better delineated than with white light. Better assessment of microvessels requires magnification (Edouard Herriot Hospital).

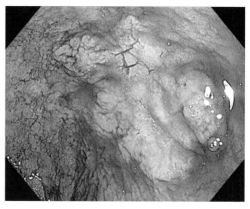

Figure 12.70 Superficial gastric carcinoma IIa–IIc: indigocarmine. Margins seen more easily for this raised lesion than with NBI (corresponds to Figures 12.68–12.69) (Edouard Herriot Hospital).

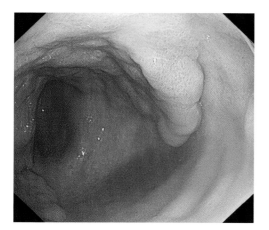

Figure 12.71 White light HRE view of an early gastric carcinoma in a background of intestinal metaplasia and atrophy (University of Amsterdam).

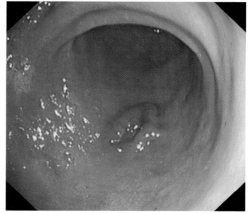

Figure 12.72 Intramucosal carcinoma, intestinal type, of the antrum. At a distance this white light view raises suspicions of a malignant appearing ulcer (corresponds to Figures 12.73–12.75) (University of Amsterdam).

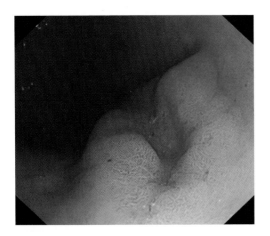

Figure 12.73 Intramucosal carcinoma, intestinal type, of the antrum. Close up white light view of the malignant appearing lesion depicted in Figure 12.72 (University of Amsterdam).

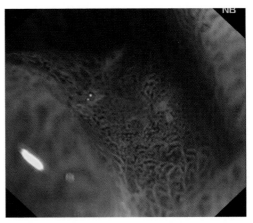

Figure 12.74 Detailed view of the center of type IIa–IIc intramucosal carcinoma of the antrum. Mesh pattern of microvessels with loss of mucosal structure predicts well-differentiated tumor and possible candidacy for ESD (University of Amsterdam).

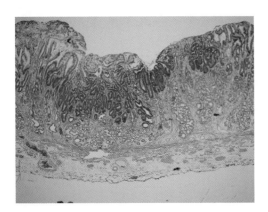

Figure 12.75 High-grade dysplasia/well-differentiated intramucosal adenocarcinoma (intestinal type). No penetration of the muscularis mucosae, confirming the optical diagnosis made in Figure 12.74 using magnification NBI (corresponds to Figures 12.72–12.74) (University of Amsterdam).

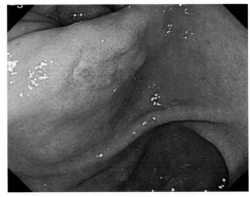

Figure 12.76 White light HRE image of small-depressed lesion in the gastric angularis suspicious for a Type 0 IIc carcinoma (corresponds to Figures 12.77–12.79) (The Jikei University School of Medicine) (copyright M. Kaise, T. Nakayoshi, H. Tajiri).

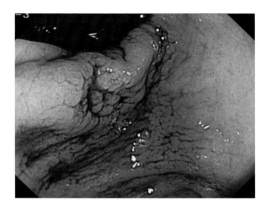

Figure 12.77 Chromoendoscopy highlights the mucosal pattern of this depressed lesion consisted of poorly differentiated carcinoma (The Jikei University School of Medicine) (copyright M. Kaise, T. Nakayoshi, H. Tajiri).

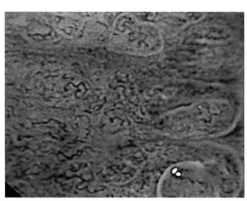

Figure 12.78 NBI magnification of this lesion reveals loss of mucosal pattern in the depressed area with abnormal microvessels in the corkscrew pattern consistent with poorly differentiated adenocarcinoma (The Jikei University School of Medicine) (copyright M. Kaise, T. Nakayoshi, H. Tajiri).

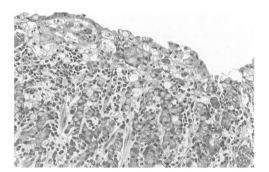

Figure 12.79 Histopathology high-power view confirms the diagnosis of poorly differentiated carcinoma predicted by the NBI analysis of the microvessel pattern (corresponds to Figures 12.76–12.78) (The Jikei University School of Medicine) (copyright M. Kaise, T. Nakayoshi, H. Tajiri).

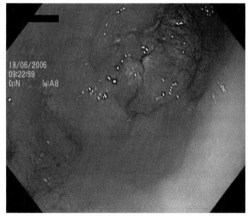

Figure 12.80 Malignant gastric ulcer in distal body, low-magnification NBI view (corresponds to Figures 12.81 and 12.82) (Hospital Sao Marcos).

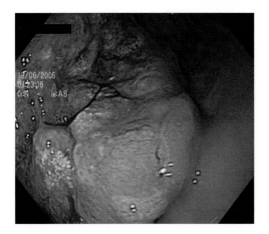

Figure 12.81 Magnified white light view of malignant gastric ulcer with irregular borders and necrotic center (Hospital Sao Marcos).

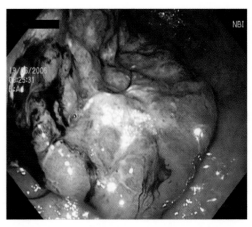

Figure 12.82 NBI magnified view of this large raised lesion that grossly suggests sm2 invasion or greater (corresponds to Figures 12.80 and 12.81) (Hospital Sao Marcos).

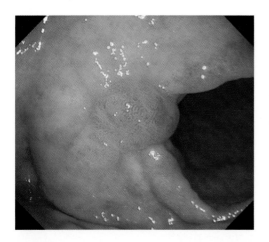

Figure 12.83 White light HRE low-magnification view of local recurrence after EMR for superficial gastric cancer (corresponds to Figures 12.84–12.86) (National Cancer Center Hospital East) (copyright M. Muto).

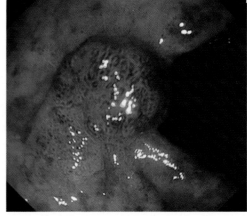

Fig. 12.84 NBI clearly shows worrisome features not apparent on white light even without magnification. This case underscores the rationale for consideration of ESD for larger superficial lesions to reduce the risk of local recurrence (National Cancer Center Hospital East) (copyright M. Muto).

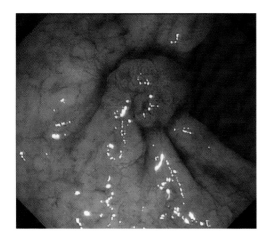

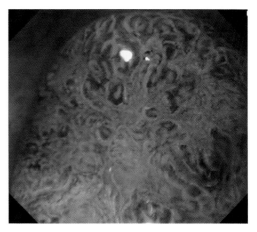

Figure 12.85 Chromoendoscopy view of local recurrence after EMR for gastric cancer (corresponds to Figures 12.83–12.86) (National Cancer Center Hospital East) (copyright M. Muto).

Figure 12.86 Magnification NBI shows both abnormal, disrupted pit pattern and abnormal vessels in this recurrent cancer (National Cancer Center Hospital East) (copyright M. Muto).

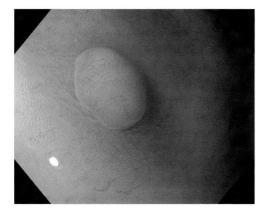

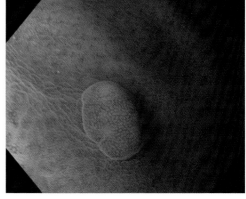

Figure 12.87 Isolated small fundic gland polyp, white light non-magnified view (NYU School of Medicine).

Figure 12.88 Isolated fundic gland polyp, low-magnification NBI view (NYU School of Medicine).

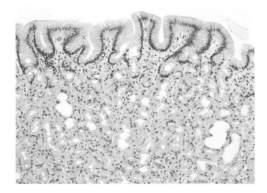

Figure 12.89 Fundic gland polyp. Oxyntic mucosa with focal cystic dilation of the glands (corresponds to Figures 12.87 and 12.88) (NYU School of Medicine).

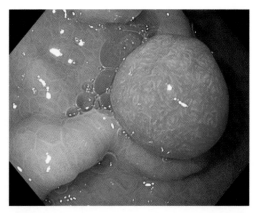

Figure 12.90 Inflammed fundic gastric polyp seen here in white light HRE view (Mayo Clinic, Jacksonville).

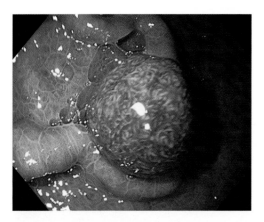

Figure 12.91 NBI view of the lesion in Figure 12.90 with clearly delineated regular pit pattern (Mayo Clinic, Jacksonville).

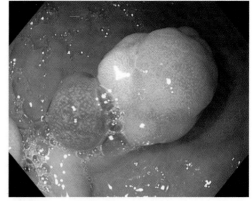

Figure 12.92 High-resolution white light image of unusual appearing fundic gland polyps in the body of the stomach of varying size and degree of inflammation (corresponds to Figure 12.93) (Mayo Clinic, Jacksonville).

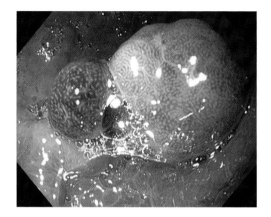

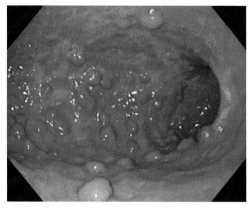

Figure 12.93 NBI of unusual appearing fundic gland polyps in the body of the stomach of varying size and degree of inflammation. Pathology confirmed this as a fundic gland polyp with hyperplastic and inflammatory fibroid polypoid features (corresponds to Figure 12.92) (Mayo Clinic, Jacksonville).

Figure 12.94 Multiple fundic gland polyps white light non-magnified view (Institut Arnault Tzanck).

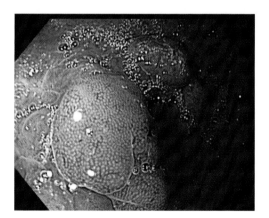

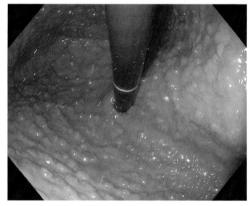

Figure 12.95 Close up view of larger fundic gland polyp with regular pit pattern well seen (corresponds to Figure 12.94) (Institut Arnault Tzanck).

Figure 12.96 White light view of multiple small sessile fundic gland polyps in familial adenomatous polyposis. Note the lack of detail of the polyp mucosa and the similar color of the polyps and gastric mucosa (corresponds to Figures 12.97–12.100) (University of Utah Health Sciences Center).

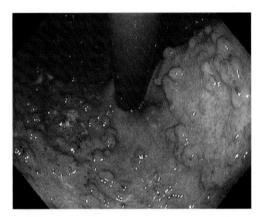

Figure 12.97 NBI view of multiple small sessile fundic gland polyps in familial adenomatous polyposis. Note that the polyps are darker than the mucosa and the polyp mucosa has a larger and more pronounced reticulated pattern (corresponds to Figures 12.96–12.100) (University of Utah Health Sciences Center).

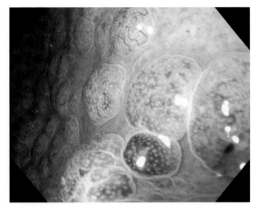

Figure 12.98 NBI magnified view of fundic land polyps. Note that the small blood vessels and pitted surface of the polyps are clearly seen (University of Utah Health Sciences Center).

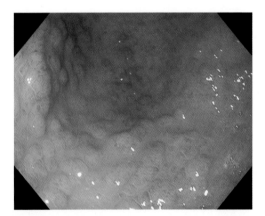

Figure 12.99 White light view of fundic gland polyps with a similar color to the gastric mucosa, a nodular appearance and scant mucosal detail (University of Utah Health Sciences Center).

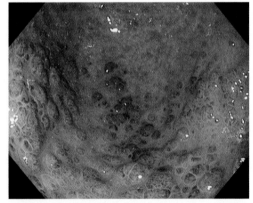

Figure 12.100 NBI view of fundic gland polyps accentuated with a darker color than the gastric mucosa, a clearly defined nodular appearance and precise mucosal detail (University of Utah Health Sciences Center).

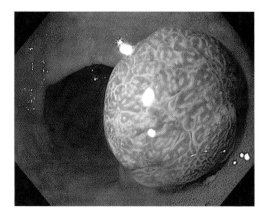

Figure 12.101 Hyperplastic antral polyp seen here in NBI low-magnification view. Note the regular round surface mucosal pattern (Edouard Herriot Hospital).

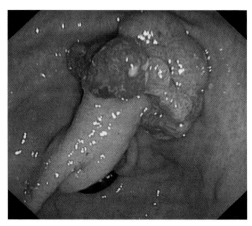

Figure 12.102 Hamartomatous polyp, indefinite for dysplasia (corresponds to Figures 12.103–12.105) (University of Amsterdam).

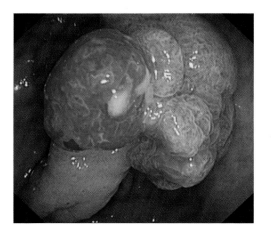

Figure 12.103 Magnified white light image of Figure 12.102, large gastric hamartomatous polyp (University of Amsterdam).

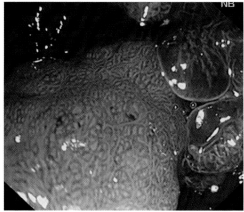

Figure 12.104 NBI magnification view highlights the transition of the mucosal patterns from the stalk to the darker more villous appearing area to the right of the image. (University of Amsterdam).

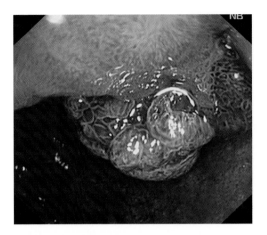

Figure 12.105 Inflamed appearing tip of the large gastric polyp (Figures 12.102–12.104) with pathologic findings indefinite for dysplasia (University of Amsterdam).

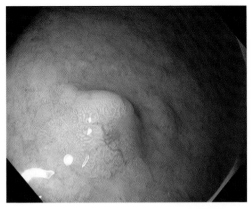

Figure 12.106 Corpus greater curvature, larger proximal and smaller distal lesion positive for carcinoid, white light HRE (University Medical Center Hamburg Eppendorf).

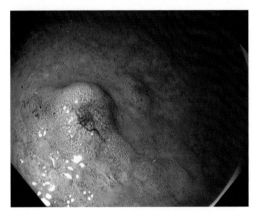

Figure 12.107 NBI HRE low-magnification view of gastric carcinoid tumors in the body, greater curvature (University Medical Center Hamburg Eppendorf).

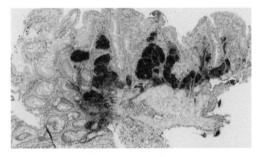

Figure 12.108 Gastric carcinoid arising in a setting of atrophic gastritis and intestinal metaplasia (corresponds to Figures 12.106 and 12.107) (University Medical Center Hamburg Eppendorf).

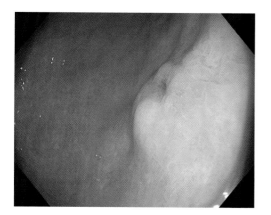

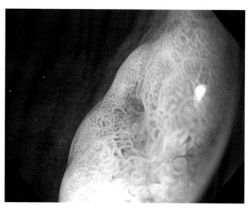

Figure 12.109 Gastric carcinoid white light low-magnification view in the antrum, posterior wall: Biopsies from the center as well as from the margin of the lesion positive for carcinoid (University Medical Center Hamburg Eppendorf).

Figure 12.110 Gastric carcinoid, close-up HRE NBI image (University Medical Center Hamburg Eppendorf).

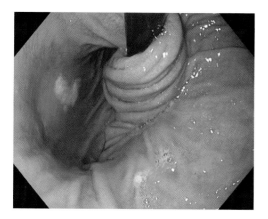

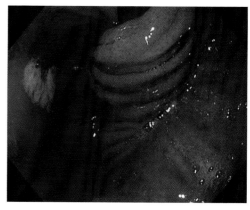

Figure 12.111 Nissen-type fundoplication, with wrap well intact in this HRE white light view (Mayo Clinic, Jacksonville).

Figure 12.112 Nissen-type fundoplication, NBI view. Note the darker appearance due to the large lumen makes NBI less useful for general use in the stomach and most appropriate for close-up magnification of suspicious lesions (Mayo Clinic, Jacksonville).

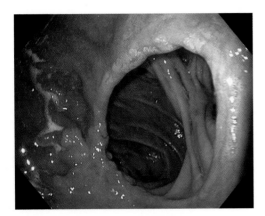

Figure 12.113 White light HRE image provides a sharp view of this gastrojejunal anastamosis. A Bilroth II gastrectomy had been performed in this patient 53 years ago for recurrent ulcers (University Medical Center Hamburg Eppendorf).

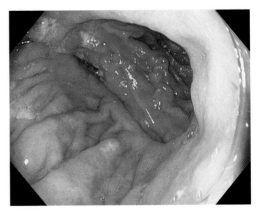

Figure 12.114 Low-magnification HRE of asymptomatic 71-year-old female 50 years following BII gastrectomy. From a distance in white light, no suspicious lesion is seen (University Medical Center Hamburg Eppendorf).

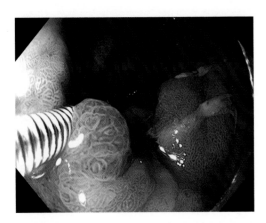

Figure 12.115 Close up with HRE and NBI of LGIN at the B-II anastomosis with 0.8 mm diameter biopsy forceps as scale. The wide sulci and irregular mucosal pattern on NBI raises the suspicion for dysplasia and allows for target biopsy of the lesion (corresponds to Figures 12.114–12.116) (University Medical Center Hamburg Eppendorf).

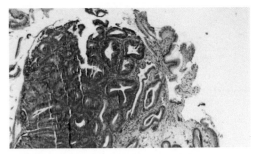

Figure 12.116 10× HE image shows LGIN in the area of a Billroth II anastomosis (University Medical Center Hamburg Eppendorf).

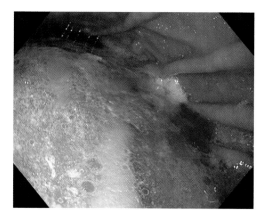

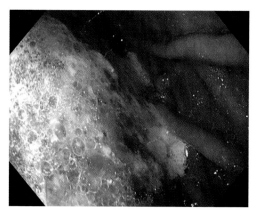

Figure 12.117 Retained contents, white light HRE, in gastric remnant after esophagectomy (Mayo Clinic, Jacksonville).

Figure 12.118 Low-magnification NBI view shows the oily remnants which now appear pink instead of yellow (corresponds to Figure 12.117) (Mayo Clinic, Jacksonville).

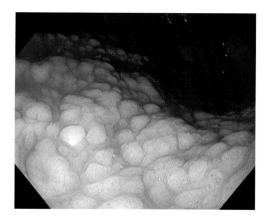

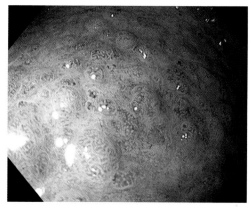

Figure 12.119 HRE low-magnification view of micronodular appearance of rare entity of collagenous gastritis (fundus) (Mayo Clinic, Jacksonville).

Figure 12.120 NBI of micronodular fundic folds in collagenous gastritis (Mayo Clinic, Jacksonville).

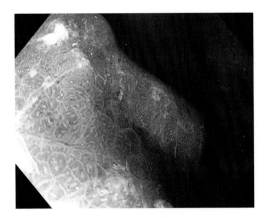

Figure 12.121 Gastric fundus in patient with MALT lymphoma following *Helicobacter pylori* eradication and 1 month of Rituxan therapy, NBI low-magnification view (NYU School of Medicine).

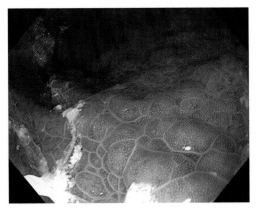

Figure 12.122 Prominent bumps and grooves in gastric body in patient with MALT lymphoma following *Helicobacter pylori* eradication and 1 month of Rituxan therapy, NBI low-magnification view (NYU School of Medicine).

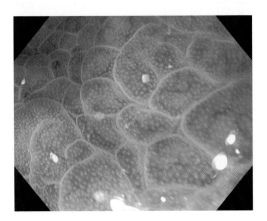

Figure 12.123 Prominent bumps and grooves in gastric body in patient with MALT lymphoma following *Helicobacter pylori* eradication and 1 month of Rituxan therapy, NBI magnification view (NYU School of Medicine).

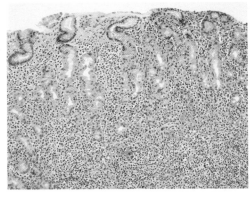

Figure 12.124 Malt lymphoma. A dense infiltrate of atypical lymphoid cells expands the mucosa and destroys gastric glands (corresponds to Figures 12.121–12.125) (NYU School of Medicine).

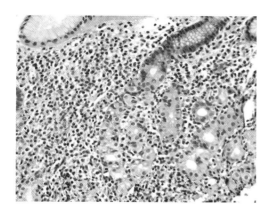

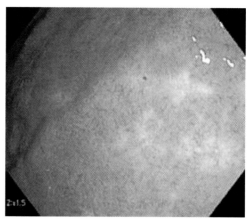

Figure 12.125 Malt lymphoma (high-power view). There is invasion and destruction of gastric gland epithelium by neoplastic lymphocytes ("lymphoepithelial lesion") (corresponds to 12.121–12.124).

Figure 12.126 White light low magnification endoscopic view of gastric MALT hyperplasia (Catholic University of the Sacred Heart).

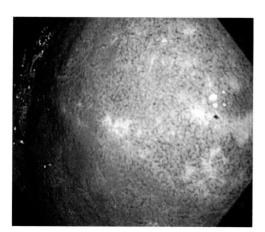

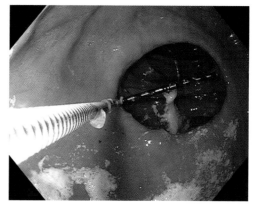

Figure 12.127 NBI low-magnification view of gastric MALT hyperplasia (corresponds to Figure 12.126) (Catholic University of the Sacred Heart).

Figure 12.128 This white light HRE image shows the use of the Olympus measuring catheter to demonstrate an enlarged gastrojejunal stoma following gastric bypass surgery (Dartmouth Medical School).

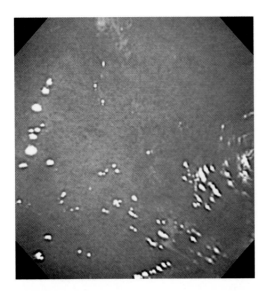 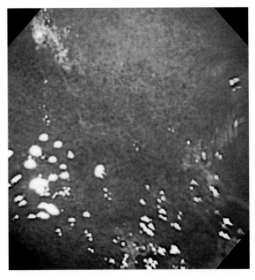

Figure 12.129 White light low-magnification image in this patient initially notable only for somewhat uneven surface contour without significant erythema or erosions (The Johns Hopkins University School of Medicine).

Figure 12.130 This magnified NBI image of the gastric antrum in this child showed non-specific congestion of vessels seen here as patches of darker areas. Biopsies revealed eosinophilic gastritis (The Johns Hopkins University School of Medicine).

ABBREVIATIONS USED

LGIN:	low-grade intraepithelial neoplasia
GAVE:	gastric antral vascular ectasia
NSAID:	nonsteroidal anti-inflammatory drug
NBI:	narrowband imaging
HRE:	high-resolution endoscopy
ESD:	endoscopic submucosal dissection
EMR:	endoscopic mucosal resection
MALT:	mucosa-associated lymphoid tissue

13 Small intestine atlas

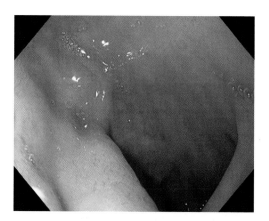

Figure 13.1 White light image of a normal duodenal bulb. The villiform architecture is indistinct (University of Utah Health Sciences Center).

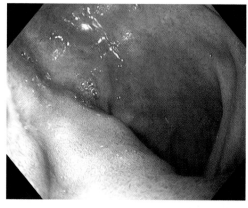

Figure 13.2 NBI low-magnification image of a normal duodenal bulb. The villiform architecture is accentuated by the NBI imaging (University of Utah Health Sciences Center).

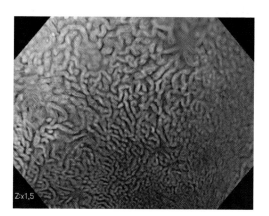

Figure 13.3 Normal mucosal appearance in the bulb NBI view 1.5× magnification (Erasmus University Hospital).

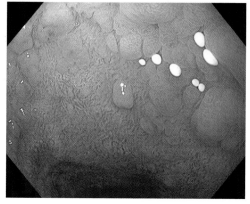

Figure 13.4 Nodular mucosa in the duodenal bulb of Bruener's glands viewed with high-resolution white light (corresponds to Figure 13.5) (Mayo Clinic, Jacksonville).

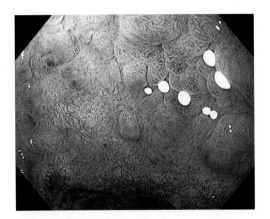

Figure 13.5 Nodular mucosa in the duo-denal bulb of Bruener's glands viewed with high-resolution narrowband image (note the white medication granules) (corresponds to Figure 13.4) (Mayo Clinic, Jacksonville).

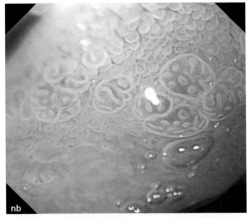

Figure 13.6 Bruener's gland hyperplasia of the duodenal bulb seen in white light HRE magnification view (Institut Arnault Tzanck).

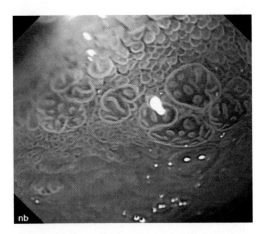

Figure 13.7 High-magnification NBI image provides excellent definition of these Bruener's glands (corresponds to Figure 13.6) (Institut Arnault Tzanck).

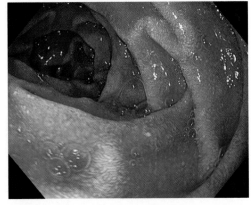

Figure 13.8 NBI light view of a normal duodenal fold. The villiform architecture is readily discernable (Medical University of South Carolina).

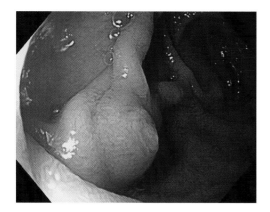

Figure 13.9 Normal major papilla (Erasmus University Hospital).

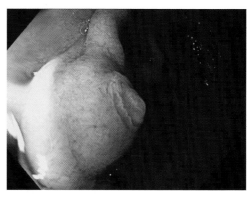

Figure 13.10 Normal major papilla under NBI low magnification (Erasmus University Hospital).

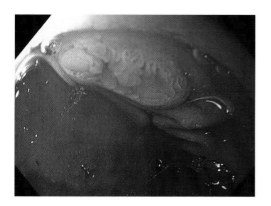

Figure 13.11 White light view of major papilla 1.2× magnification. Duodenoscope NBI HDTV not currently available, though such high definition of ampulla could one day facilitate ERCP (NYU School of Medicine).

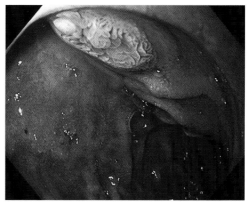

Figure 13.12 NBI non-magnification view of normal major papilla (NYU School of Medicine).

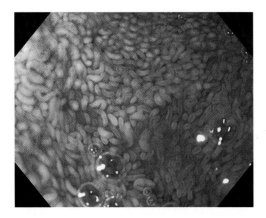

Figure 13.13 NBI HRE 1.5× magnification view of normal duodenal villi (NYU School of Medicine).

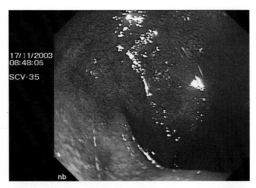

Figure 13.14 Bile appears red under NBI light (Institut Arnault Tzanck).

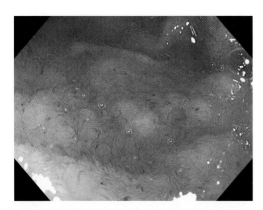

Figure 13.15 Normal ileum with bumpy lymphoid tissue and clearly discernable villi well visualized on low-magnification NBI view. In addition to the thin brownish superficial capillaries, one can appreciate some deeper vessels that appear green, such as one at the top middle of the photograph (NYU School of Medicine).

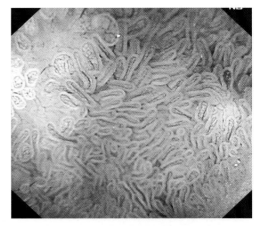

Figure 13.16 NBI with magnification of terminal ileal villi showing capillary loops and plexuses within individual villi (St. Mark's Hospital).

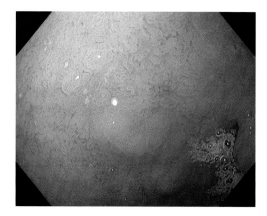

Figure 13.17 Subtle inflammation of duodenal bulb on white light non-magnified view (NYU School of Medicine).

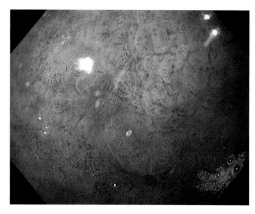

Figure 13.18 Subtle erosions and inflammation in duodenal bulb indicated on NBI non-magnified view. The contrast under NBI between the dark inflamed mucosa and the white erosion may make subtle findings such at these easier to detect (corresponds to Figure 13.17) (NYU School of Medicine).

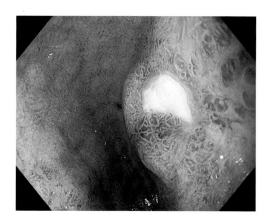

Figure 13.19 This bulb ulcer was found in a patient taking baby aspirin following one episode of melena without abdominal pain. It is not known whether NBI will enhance detection of subtle stigmata. This HRE image clearly defines this ulcer as clean based (NYU School of Medicine).

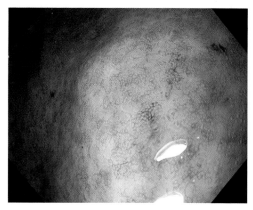

Figure 13.20 The antrum of the patient in Figure 13.19 shows prominent lymphoid follicles and the histopathology confirmed active *Helicobacter pylori* gastritis (NYU School of Medicine).

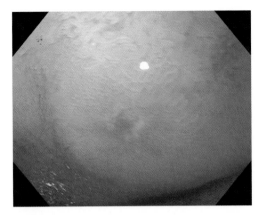

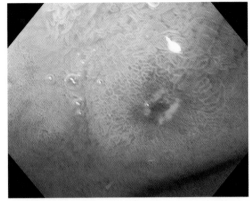

Figure 13.21 Duodenal erosion faintly visible on white light view seen here in 1.5× magnification (NYU School of Medicine).

Figure 13.22 Small duodenal erosion seen clearly with low-magnification NBI (NYU School of Medicine).

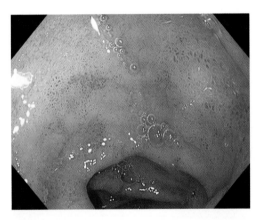

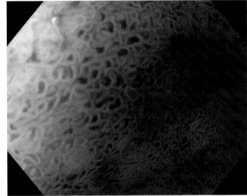

Figure 13.23 Moderate peptic duodenitis under white light low magnification (NYU School of Medicine).

Figure 13.24 Magnified NBI view of moderate duodenitis of the bulb (NYU School of Medicine).

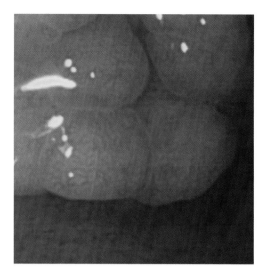

Figure 13.25 Duodenal bulb hyperplastic polyp; white light low magnification (Catholic University of the Sacred Heart).

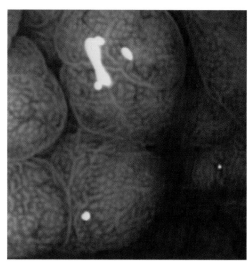

Figure 13.26 NBI view of gastric polyp located in the duodenal bulb. Regular gastric-type pit pattern seen well (Catholic University of the Sacred Heart).

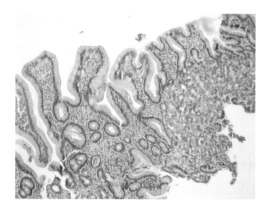

Figure 13.27 Oxyntic-type gastric crypts in the lamina propria (bottom right) and the lack of goblet and Paneth cells in the superficial epithelium are consistent with fundic-type gastric heterotopic epithelium (corresponds to Figures 13.25 and 13.26). (Catholic University of the Sacred Heart).

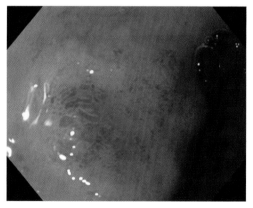

Figure 13.28 This duodenal red slightly raised area here seen in low-magnification white light might be mistaken for an area of duodenitis; however, note the irregularity of the vessels in comparison to the image of duodenitis in Figure 13.23 above (corresponds to Figures 13.29 and 13.30) (Edouard Herriot Hospital).

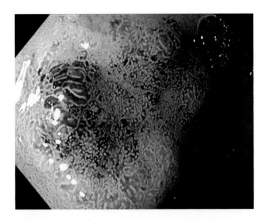

Figure 13.29 On NBI, the gyrus mucosal surface pattern and vascular pattern more readily identify this lesion as an adenoma (corresponds to Figures 13.28–13.30). (Edouard Herriot Hospital).

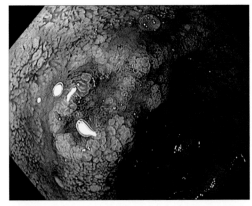

Figure 13.30 Indigocarmine view of the same lesion; NBI appears to provide better delineation of this adenoma (Edouard Herriot Hospital).

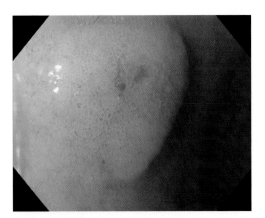

Figure 13.31 Flat duodenal polyp; pathology revealed undifferentiated adenocarcinoma with invasion of the submucosa (HRE white light) (University Medical Center Hamburg Eppendorf).

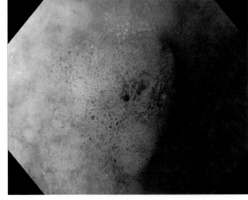

Figure 13.32 NBI low-magnification view of this flat duodenal bulb adenocarcinoma highlights abnormal surface contour and irregular vessels (University Medical Center Hamburg Eppendorf).

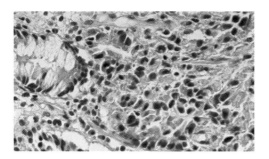

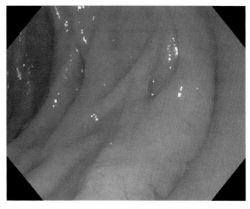

Figure 13.33 Poorly differentiated duodenal adenocarcinoma (corresponds to Figures 13.31 and 13.32) (University Medical Center Hamburg Eppendorf).

Figure 13.34 Duodenal adenoma detected as an irregular fold on white light low magnification (Edouard Herriot Hospital).

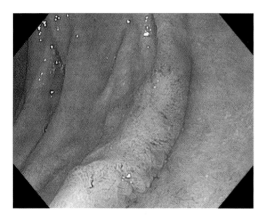

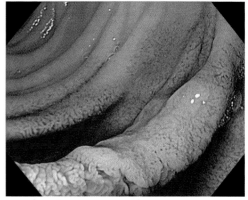

Figure 13.35 NBI low magnification view of duodenal adenoma: the lesion appears whitish whereas the normal background is pink. Easier to be detected than white light (corresponds to Figures 13.34 and 13.36) (Edouard Herriot Hospital).

Figure 13.36 Indigo carmine image provides similar image to the NBI; NBI appears as easier replacement to chromoendoscopy (Edouard Herriot Hospital).

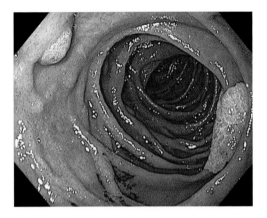

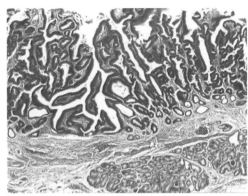

Figure 13.37 Low-magnification NBI image of duodenal adenoma opposite to the papilla. Both papilla and polyp appear gray and normal duodenal mucosa appears pink (Edouard Herriot Hospital).

Figure 13.38 Duodenal adenoma. The normal mucosa is replaced by a tubulo-villous proliferation lined by hyperchromatic dysplastic epithelium (corresponds to Figure 13.37) (Edouard Herriot Hospital).

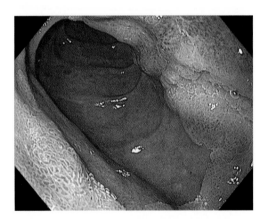

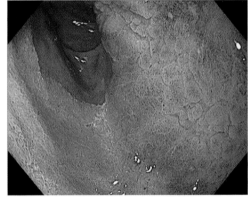

Figure 13.39 Extensive circumferential duodenal adenoma from the pylorus to D3. Lower margin in D3 which is very clearly discerned using NBI with low magnification (Edouard Herriot Hospital).

Figure 13.40 NBI view of lower end of adenoma; notice the irregular surface pattern and vasculature highlighted by the NBI (corresponds to Figures 13.39–13.44) (Edouard Herriot Hospital) .

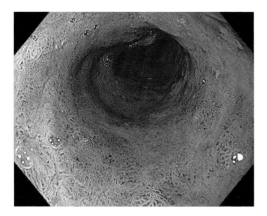

Figure 13.41 NBI low-magnification view of middle of this lateral spreading adenoma (corresponds to Figures 13.39–13.44) (Edouard Herriot Hospital).

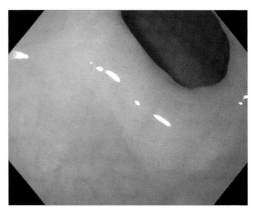

Figure 13.42 Extensive duodenal adenoma from the pylorus to D3. View from the antrum: irregular pattern on the pylorus. White light non-magnified image (Edouard Herriot Hospital).

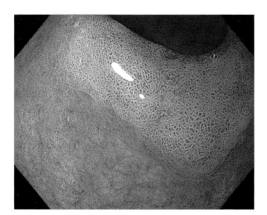

Figure 13.43 Low-magnification NBI view from the antrum greatly accentuates the margin of the lesion compared to white light view shown in Figure 13.42 (Edouard Herriot Hospital).

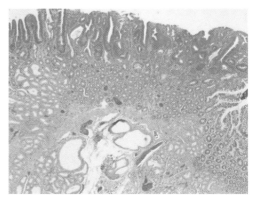

Figure 13.44 Duodenal adenoma. Dysplastic epithelium has replaced the duodenal epithelium in the upper half of the mucosa and spread widely, forming an extensive flat carpet of dysplasia (corresponds to Figures 13.39–13.43) (Edouard Herriot Hospital).

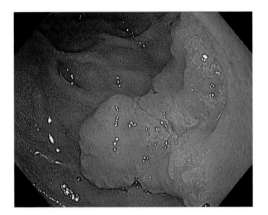

Figure 13.45 White light low-magnification HRE view of large sessile duodenal adenoma (Edouard Herriot Hospital).

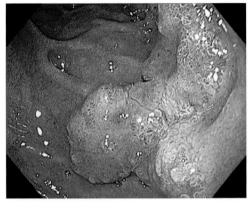

Figure 13.46 NBI low-magnification view of large sessile duodenal adenoma: better delineation and characterization with NBI (Edouard Herriot Hospital).

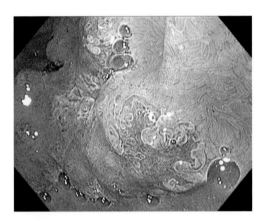

Figure 13.47 This closer view with the same magnification illustrates the physical zoom property of the HDTV endoscopy; the image sharpness is not reduced when the scope tip is pushed closer to the lesion (corresponds to Figures 13.45 and 13.46) (Edouard Herriot Hospital).

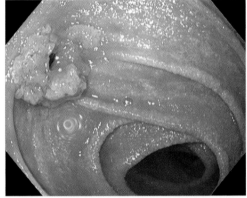

Figure 13.48 Bile duct adenoma with high-grade dysplasia seen here with high-resolution white light (note yellow colored bile) (corresponds to Figures 13.49–13.51) (Mayo Clinic, Jacksonville).

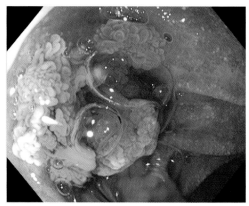

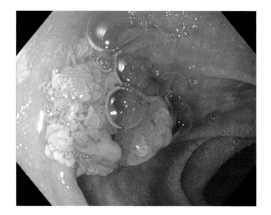

Figure 13.49 Close-up high-resolution white light image of bile duct adenoma with high-grade dysplasia (note yellow colored bile) (Mayo Clinic, Jacksonville).

Figure 13.50 Close-up image of bile duct adenoma with high-grade dysplasia viewed with high-resolution narrow band image (note red colored bile) (Mayo Clinic, Jacksonville).

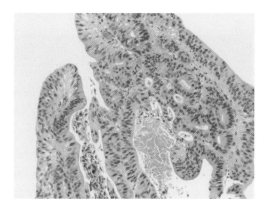

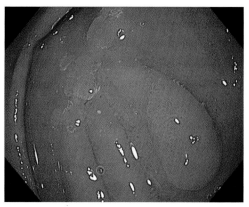

Figure 13.51 Histologic image of bile duct adenoma with high-grade dysplasia (corresponds to Figures 13.48–13.50) (Mayo Clinic, Jacksonville).

Figure 13.52 White light low-magnification view of FAP: duodenal lesions (corresponds to Figures 13.53–13.55) (Edouard Herriot Hospital).

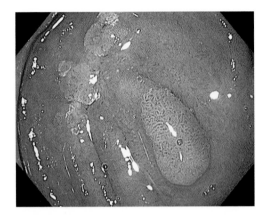

Figure 13.53 NBI image of FAP: duodenal lesions which appear whitish on pink background. Better delineation and characterization than with white light (corresponds to Figures 13.52–13.55) (Edouard Herriot Hospital).

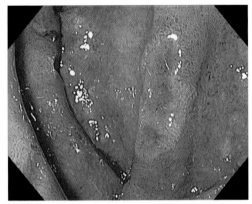

Figure 13.54 Varying appearance of FAP: large grey-white lesion in the duodenum under NBI, low-magnification (Edouard Herriot Hospital).

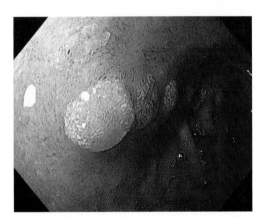

Figure 13.55 FAP: several adenomas easily detected with NBI, here with a white appearance. Indigocarmine is not necessary for identification or assessment of borders (Edouard Herriot Hospital).

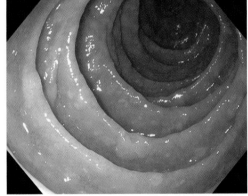

Figure 13.56 White light view of numerous small adenomas in D3 in a patient with FAP (corresponds to Figure 13.57) (University of Utah Health Sciences Center).

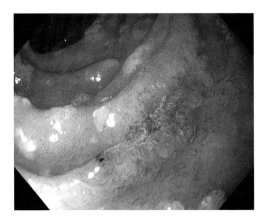

Figure 13.57 Magnification NBI view in this patient clearly defines the lesions as sessile adenomas (corresponds to Figure 13.56) (University of Utah Health Sciences Center).

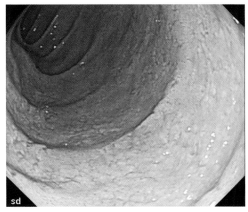

Figure 13.58 Complete villous atrophy, HRE white light low-magnification view (Institut Arnault Tzanck).

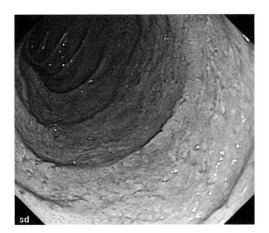

Figure 13.59 Completely flattened villi seen on NBI low-magnification view. Histopathology confirmed endoscopic impression of total villous atrophy (corresponds to Figures 13.58) (Institut Arnault Tzanck).

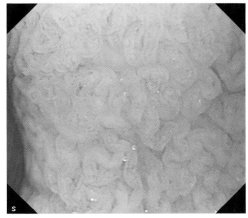

Figure 13.60 Partial villous atrophy, white light HRE magnification view (corresponds to Figure 13.61) (Institut Arnault Tzanck).

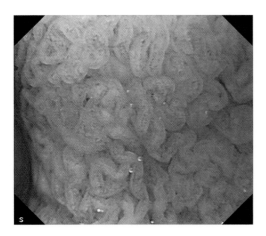

Figure 13.61 Partial villous atrophy, magnified NBI image (corresponds to Figure 13.60) (Institut Arnault Tzanck).

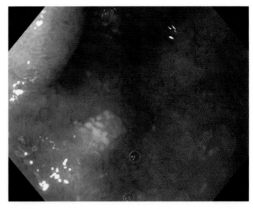

Figure 13.62 NBI 1.5× magnified view of jejunal lymphangiectasia in an efferent limb of a gastrojejunostomy (NYU School of Medicine).

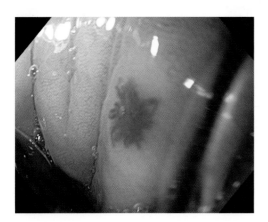

Figure 13.63 Arterio-vascular malformation viewed with high-resolution white light (Mayo Clinic, Jacksonville).

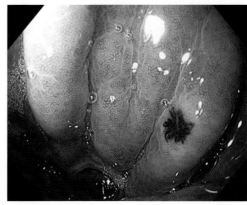

Figure 13.64 Arterio-vascular malformation viewed with high-resolution narrowband image (Mayo Clinic, Jacksonville).

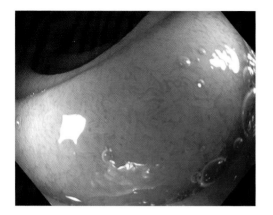

Figure 13.65 Duodenal angioectasia with subtle appearance well appreciated using HRE, white light (Institut Arnault Tzanck).

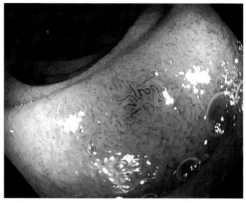

Figure 13.66 NBI view of the same lesion clearly enhances the detection of this vascular abnormality (Institut Arnault Tzanck).

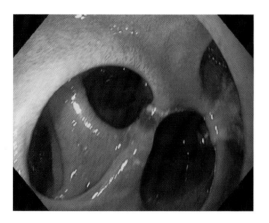

Figure 13.67 Multiple large duodenal diverticula, white light low-magnification view (Institut Arnault Tzanck).

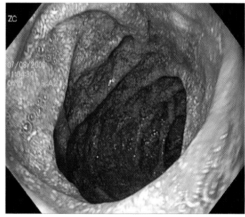

Figure 13.68 Small bowel Whipple's disease with whitish plaque-like patches, white light low-magnification view (corresponds to Figures 13.69–13.71) (Hospital Sao Marcos).

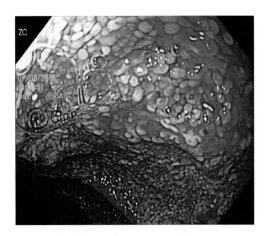

Figure 13.69 NBI view of small bowel Whipple's disease; the contrast highlights the whitish plaque-like patches (corresponds to Figures 13.68–13.71) (Hospital Sao Marcos).

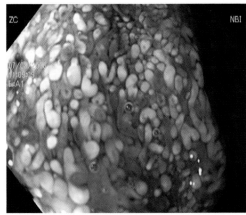

Figure 13.70 NBI 1.5× magnification of small bowel Whipple's disease highlighting the whitish plaque-like patches (Hospital Sao Marcos).

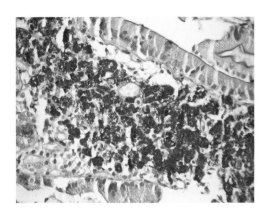

Figure 13.71 Histological image of Whipple's disease showing PAS positive macrophages in lamina propria (Hospital Sao Marcos).

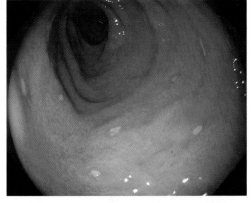

Figure 13.72 White light low-magnification image of multiple small ulcers of the distal ileum due to NSAIDs. Note the reddened borders of the punctuate white lesions indicating that these are ulcerations; in NBI in Figure 13.73, these appear as dark rings providing striking contrast to the erosions within (University of Utah Health Sciences Center).

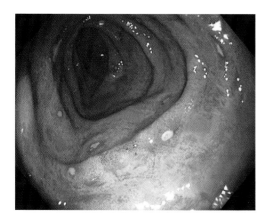

Figure 13.73 NBI low-magnification image of distal ileal ulcers due to NSAIDs (corresponds to Figures 13.72) (University of Utah Health Sciences Center).

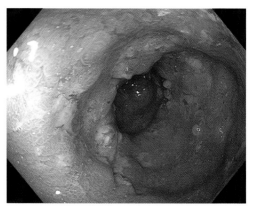

Figure 13.74 White light view depicts multifocal abnormal ileal mucosa in Crohn's disease. This appearance is more diffuse than the punctuate NSAID associated ileal ulcers depicted in Figures 13.72 and 13.73. The degree of mucosal irregularity stands in considerable contrast to the bumpy lymphoid tissue of the normal ileum (Figure 13.15) (Institut Arnault Tzanck).

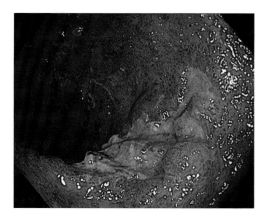

Figure 13.75 NBI image clearly delineates a large ileal Crohn's ulcer along with diffuse inflammation of the surrounding tissue (Institut Arnault Tzanck).

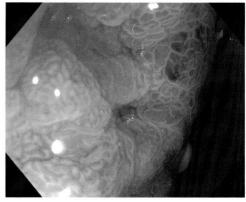

Figure 13.76 Aphthous ulcer in terminal ileum in Crohn's disease. The heaped-up epithelium surrounds a tiny ulcer. NBI view (Mount Sinai School of Medicine).

ABBREVIATIONS USED

ERCP: endoscopic retrograde cholangiopancreatography
FAP: familial adenomatous polyposis
HDTV: high-definition TV
HRE: high-resolution endoscopy
NBI: narrowband imaging
NSAIDs: non-steroidal anti-inflammatory drugs
PAS: *p*-aminosalicylic acid

Colon atlas

14

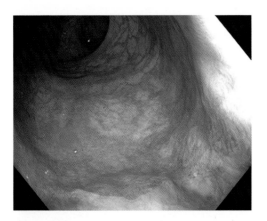

Figure 14.1 HRE white light low-magnification view of normal rectum with clear demarcation of the dentate line (NYU School of Medicine).

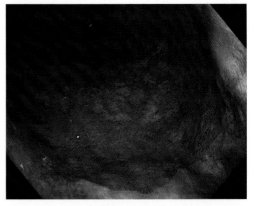

Figure 14.2 Similar view of normal rectum seen here in low-magnification NBI (NYU School of Medicine).

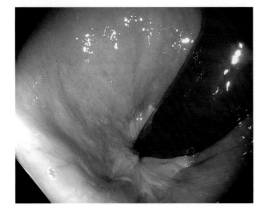

Figure 14.3 Retroflexed view of a normal rectum. Note the sharp demarcation of the dentate line (University of Utah Health Sciences Center).

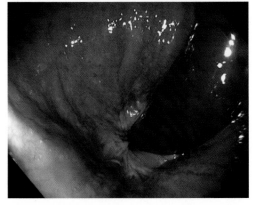

Figure 14.4 Retroflexed NBI view of a normal rectum. Note the sharp demarcation of the dentate line (University of Utah Health Sciences Center).

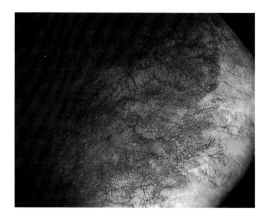

Figure 14.5 NBI view clearly demarcating dentate line (NYU School of Medicine).

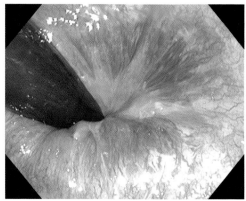

Figure 14.6 White light retroflex view of distal rectum (NYU School of Medicine).

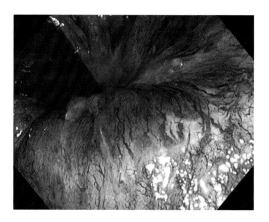

Figure 14.7 NBI rectal retroflex view highlights prominent vascular pattern (NYU School of Medicine).

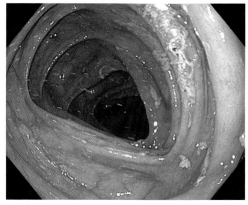

Figure 14.8 Normal colon with bilious stool, HRE (Mayo Clinic, Jacksonville).

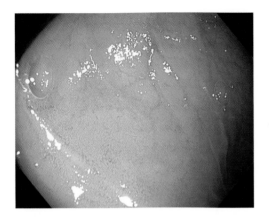

Figure 14.9 White light view of normal colon (NYU School of Medicine).

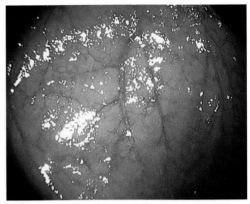

Figure 14.10 NBI non-magnified view of normal colon demonstrates vascular pattern poorly seen on white light view of Figure 14.9 (NYU School of Medicine).

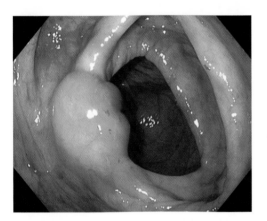

Figure 14.11 Ileocecal valve with bilious stool, HRE white light view (Mayo Clinic, Jacksonville).

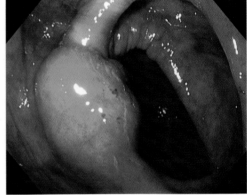

Figure 14.12 Ileocecal valve with bilious stool, NBI low-magnification image (Mayo Clinic, Jacksonville).

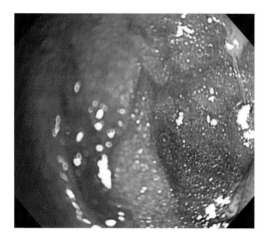

Figure 14.13 Post-polypectomy from ileocecal valve, submucosal fat viewed under white light (Lenox Hill Hospital).

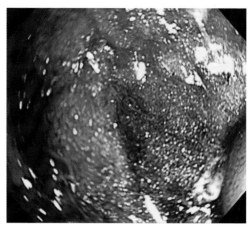

Figure 14.14 NBI image has no advantage in viewing submucosal fat (Lenox Hill Hospital).

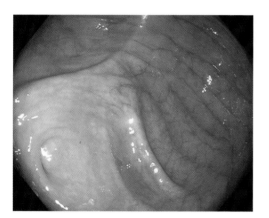

Figure 14.15 Normal appendiceal orifice viewed with HRE white light (University of Utah Health Sciences Center).

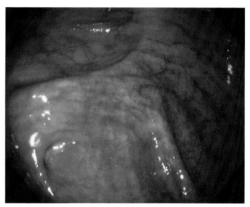

Figure 14.16 Normal appendiceal orifice viewed with NBI light (University of Utah Health Sciences Center).

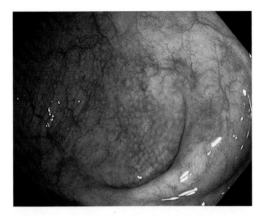

Figure 14.17 Non-magnified view of normal appendiceal orifice with prominent lymphoid tissue highlighted with NBI (NYU School of Medicine).

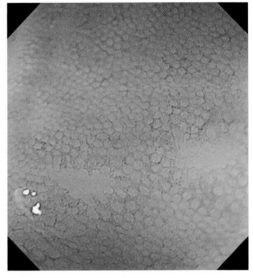

Figure 14.18 Lymphoid follicles in cecum seen here on white light magnified view (St. Mark's Hospital).

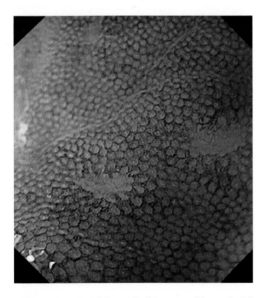

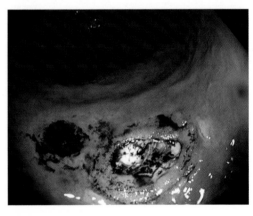

Figure 14.20 NBI image post-biopsy (University of Utah Health Sciences Center).

Figure 14.19 Magnified image of lymphoid follicles in cecum. Note honeycomb capillary plexuses around pits in normal mucosa seen well with NBI (corresponds to Figure 14.18) (St. Mark's Hospital).

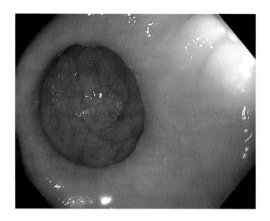

Figure 14.21 Large diverticulum shown in HRE white light view (NYU School of Medicine).

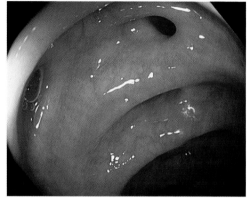

Figure 14.22 HRE white light non-magnified view of a diverticulum (NYU School of Medicine).

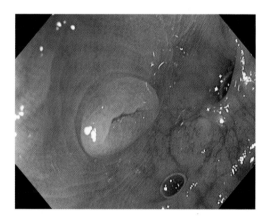

Figure 14.23 Everted diverticulum with NBI image confirming normal colon pit pattern to avoid mistaken identification as a polyp (NYU School of Medicine).

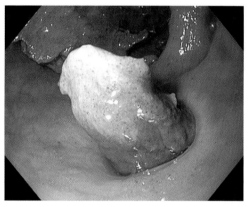

Figure 14.24 Residual stool within diverticulum, white light view (corresponds to Figure 14.25) (NYU School of Medicine).

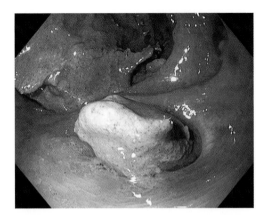

Figure 14.25 NBI image of residual stool lodged in a diverticulum. Stool appears pink in NBI (corresponds to Figure 14.24) (NYU School of Medicine).

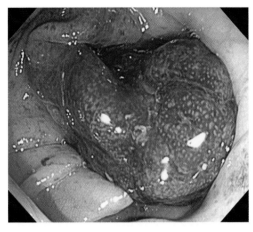

Figure 14.26 Polypoid red fold of diverticular disease – note normal pit pattern (Mount Sinai School of Medicine).

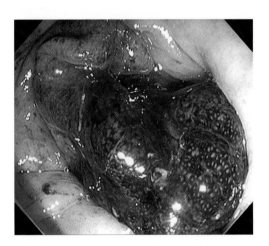

Figure 14.27 Polypoid red fold of diverticular disease – note normal pit pattern (corresponds to Figure 14.26) (NBI image) (Mount Sinai School of Medicine).

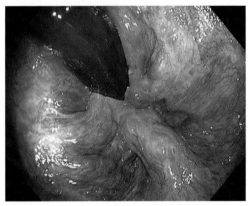

Figure 14.28 Internal hemorrhoids, retroflexion white light view (corresponds to Figure 14.29) (NYU School of Medicine).

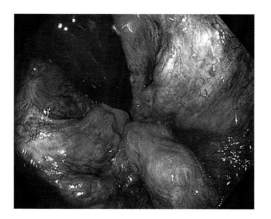

Figure 14.29 NBI image of internal hemorrhoids as seen in retroflexion (corresponds to
Figure 14.28) (NYU School of Medicine).

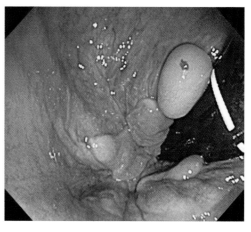

Figure 14.30 Retroflexed view in rectum
of hypertrophied anal papilla (Mount Sinai
School of Medicine).

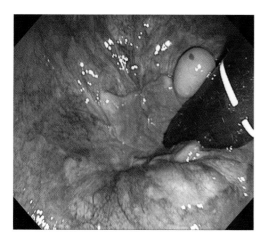

Figure 14.31 Retroflexed view in rectum of
hypertrophied anal papilla (NBI image)
(corresponds to Figure 14.30) (Mount Sinai
School of Medicine).

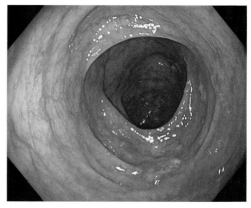

Figure 14.32 Residual feces in the descending colon viewed with white light (corresponds to Figure 14.33) (University of Utah
Health Sciences Center).

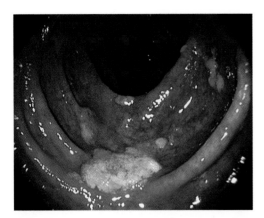

Figure 14.33 Residual feces in the descending colon seen with NBI light as pink in color (corresponds to Figure 14.32) (University of Utah Health Sciences Center).

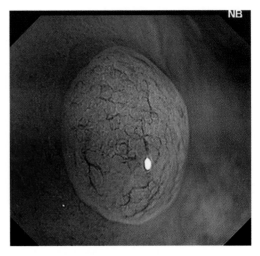

Figure 14.34 Magnified NBI image of hyperplastic polyp showing fine vessels and type 2 pit pattern (St. Mark's Hospital).

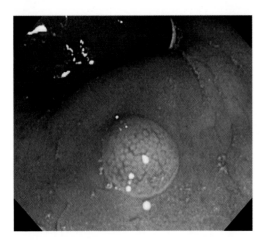

Figure 14.35 Hyperplastic appearing pit pattern on NBI non-magnified view of rectal polyp, Q180 non-high definition scope which still has NBI capability (NYU School of Medicine).

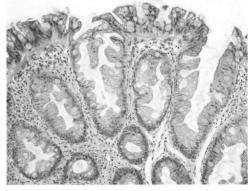

Figure 14.36 Hyperplastic polyp corresponding to Figure 14.35. Surface and gland epithelium, composed of tall cells with small basal nuclei and eosinophilic cytoplasm with mucin droplets, is thrown into papillary folds giving glands a serrated appearance (NYU School of Medicine).

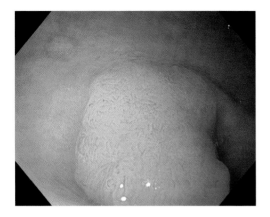

Figure 14.37 Rectal polyp under white light (Lenox Hill Hospital).

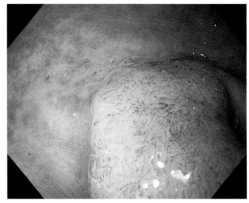

Figure 14.38 Irregular vascular pattern is more evident on rectal polyp under NBI (corresponds to Figure 14.37) (Lenox Hill Hospital).

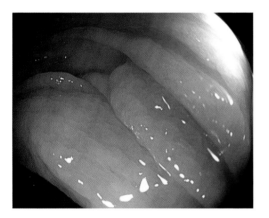

Figure 14.39 Small hyperplastic polyp in the transverse colon in white light, low magnification (Indiana University School of Medicine).

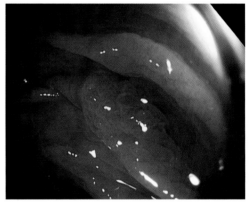

Figure 14.40 NBI image of small hyperplastic transverse colon polyp – type 1 pits (Indiana University School of Medicine).

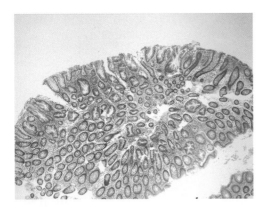

Figure 14.41 Small proximal colon hyperplastic polyp in low power (corresponds to Figures 14.39 and 14.40) (Indiana University School of Medicine).

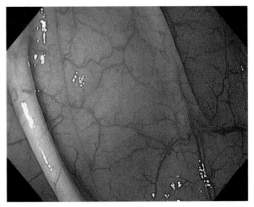

Figure 14.42 White light image fails to demonstrate a polyp (Edouard Herriot Hospital).

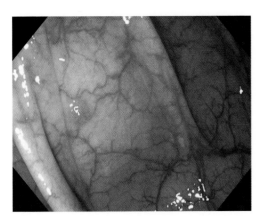

Figure 14.43 NBI view of Figure 14.42 reveals a tiny hyperplastic polyp seen only with NBI: red-brown in color (Edouard Herriot Hospital).

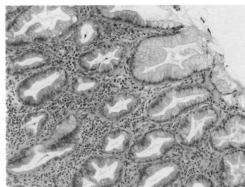

Figure 14.44 Hyperplastic polyp. Gland lumens appear stellate in histological section and are lined by bland mucinous epithelium (corresponds to Figures 14.42 and 14.43) (Edouard Herriot Hospital).

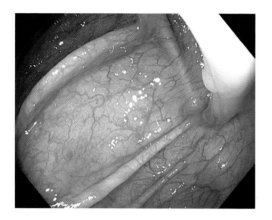

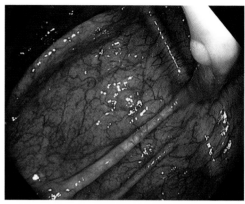

Figure 14.45 Small polyp on fold in upper right side of photo barely visible even on high-resolution white light view (NYU School of Medicine).

Figure 14.46 The same small polyp easily identified on NBI low-magnification view (NYU School of Medicine).

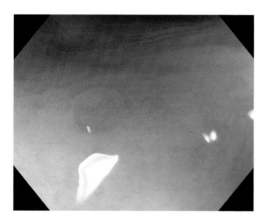

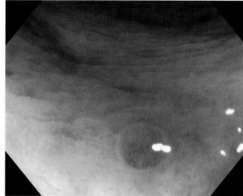

Figure 14.47 Barely discernable 1 mm rectal polyp seen with white light (University of Utah Health Sciences Center).

Figure 14.48 Clearly discernable 1 mm rectal polyp seen with NBI light with the characteristic pitted appearance of a hyperplastic polyp (University of Utah Health Sciences Center).

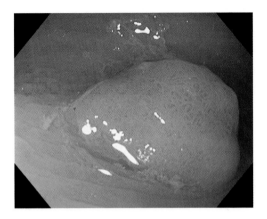

Figure 14.49 White light view of sessile polyp (NYU School of Medicine).

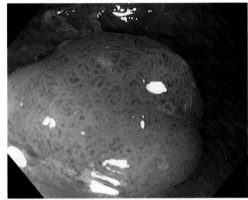

Figure 14.50 NBI image of adenoma – note high clusters of brown vessels (NYU School of Medicine).

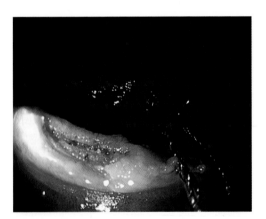

Figure 14.51 Post-polypectomy performed under NBI. Clear margins well visualized (NYU School of Medicine).

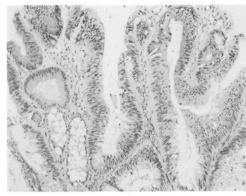

Figure 14.52 Tubulovillous adenoma with low-grade dysplasia. Glands and villi are lined by mucin-depleted cells with enlarged stratified hyperchromatic nuclei which contrast with entrapped normal glands (bottom left) (corresponds to 14.49–14.51) (NYU School of Medicine).

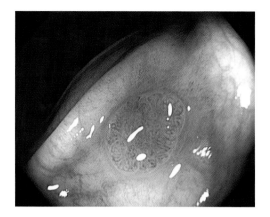

Figure 14.53 Tubular adenoma with type 3L pits. NBI low-magnification view. Note also the well-demarcated margins (Indiana University School of Medicine).

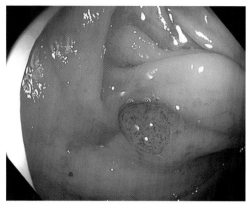

Figure 14.54 White light HRE suggests adenoma vs. inflammatory polyp in this patient with a history of malignant melanoma (corresponds to Figures 14.55 and 14.56) (NYU School of Medicine).

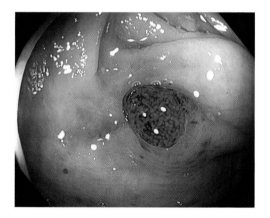

Figure 14.55 NBI magnification view of this small polyp provides extremely precise determination of its adenomatous pit pattern and vascularity, and pathology confirmed it to be a tubular adenoma (NYU School of Medicine).

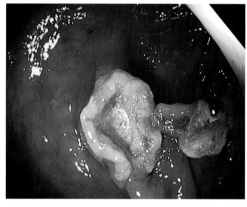

Figure 14.56 NBI image following polypectomy clearly indicates complete removal of polyp tissue (corresponds to Figures 14.54–14.55) (NYU School of Medicine).

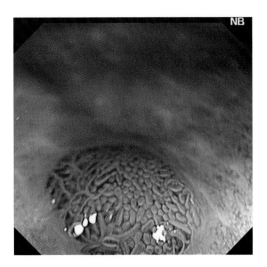

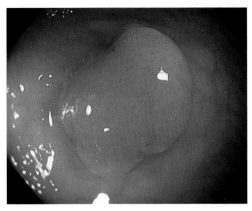

Figure 14.58 White light view of sigmoid colon tubular adenoma with low-grade dysplasia (corresponds to Figures 14.59 and 14.60) (Indiana University School of Medicine).

Figure 14.57 Magnified NBI image of a 3mm mildly dysplastic tubular adenoma with type 3L pit pattern (St. Mark's Hospital).

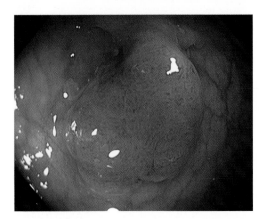

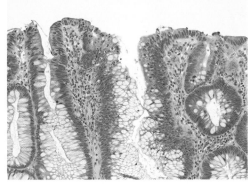

Figure 14.59 NBI image of sigmoid colon tubular adenoma with low-grade dysplasia – 3L pits (Indiana University School of Medicine).

Figure 14.60 Tubular adenoma with low-grade dysplasia, high-power view (corresponds to Figures 14.58 and 14.59) (Indiana University School of Medicine).

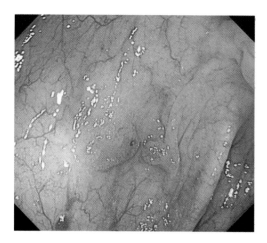

Figure 14.61 Depressed type lesion (IIc + IIa) 9 mm in size, transverse colon. The lesion is identified by a tiny oozing during standard endoscopy (Sano Hospital) (copyright Y. Sano).

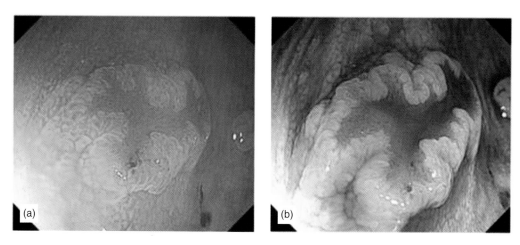

(a)

(b)

Figure 14.62 (a) Ordinary view, magnified showing central depression. (b) Indigo carmine dye spraying view. Pit pattern is not well recognized in either view (corresponds to Figures 14.61–14.65) (Sano Hospital) (copyright Y. Sano).

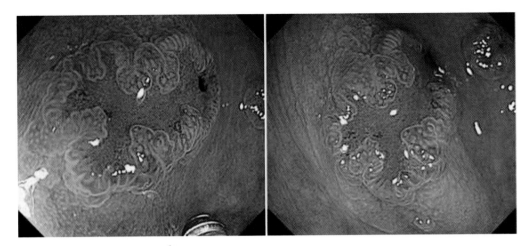

Figure 14.63 NBI colonoscopy with magnification. Kudo's IIIs pit pattern is observed clearly without dye spraying (Sano Hospital) (corresponds to Figures 14.61–14.65) (copyright Y. Sano).

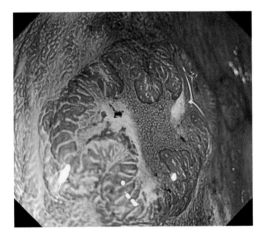

Figure 14.64 Crystal violet staining. Kudo's IIIs pit pattern is observed clearly same as NBI colonoscopy (Sano Hospital) (copyright Y. Sano).

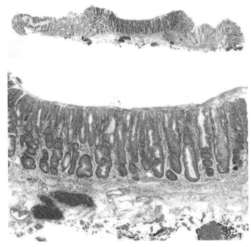

Figure 14.65 Pathological findings: adenoma with high-grade dysplasia (Sano Hospital) (copyright Y. Sano).

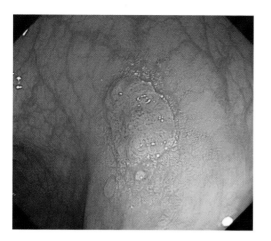

Figure 14.66 Depressed type lesion (IIa + IIc). The lesion is identified by a tiny oozing and white spots surrounding lesion during standard endoscopy (Sano Hospital) (copyright Y. Sano).

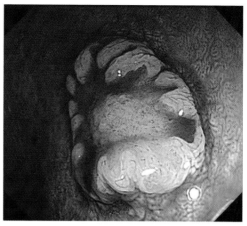

Figure 14.67 Indigo carmine dye spraying view. Pit pattern is not well recognized due to dense mucous (Sano Hospital) (copyright Y. Sano).

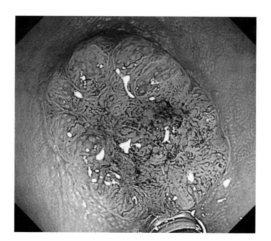

Figure 14.68 NBI colonoscopy with magnification. Sano capillary pattern type III is observed clearly without dye spraying (corresponds to Figures 14.66–14.69) (Sano Hospital) (copyright Y. Sano).

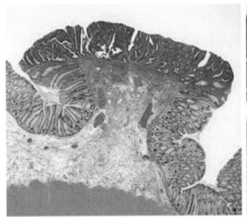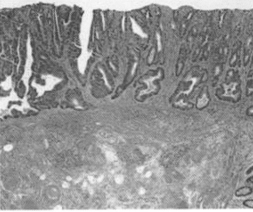

Figure 14.69 Well-differentiated intramucosal adenocarcinoma without lymphatic, vascular or neural invasion (corresponds to Figures 14.66–14.68) (Sano Hospital) (copyright Y. Sano).

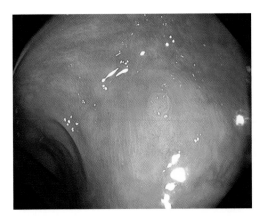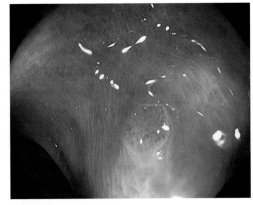

Figure 14.70 Tiny polyp seen on white light non-magnified view (NYU School of Medicine).

Figure 14.71 Adenoma pattern and well-demarcated borders evident on low-magnification NBI view (NYU School of Medicine).

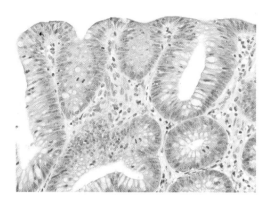

Figure 14.72 Tubular adenoma with low-grade dysplasia. Epithelial cells of the glands and surface are crowded with enlarged, stratified hyperchromatic nuclei and an increased nuclear:cytoplasmic ratio (corresponds to Figures 14.70 and 14.71) (NYU School of Medicine).

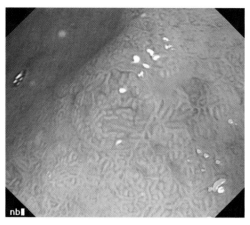

Figure 14.73 White light HRE low magnification of flat adenoma (Institut Arnault Tzanck).

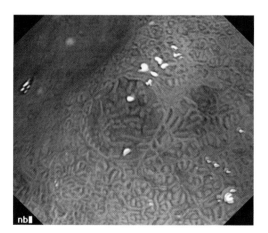

Figure 14.74 NBI image of the same lesions as Figure 14.73 (Institut Arnault Tzanck).

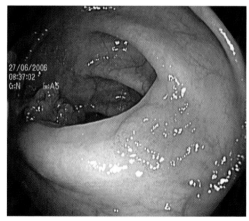

Figure 14.75 Adenomatous polyp with low-grade dysplasia in sigmoid colon (corresponds to Figures 14.76–14.80) (Hospital Sao Marcos).

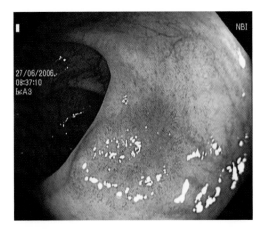

Figure 14.76 Low-grade dysplasia adenomatous polyp, with NBI high-lightened borders (corresponds to Figures 14.75–14.80) (Hospital Sao Marcos).

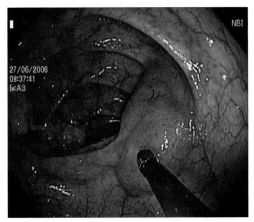

Figure 14.77 Submucosal injection previous to polypectomy (Hospital Sao Marcos).

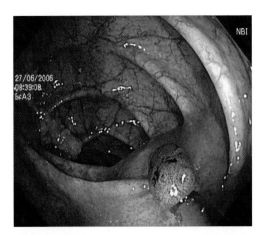

Figure 14.78 Polypectomy image with NBI (Hospital Sao Marcos).

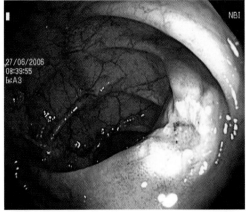

Figure 14.79 Polypectomy scar (Hospital Sao Marcos).

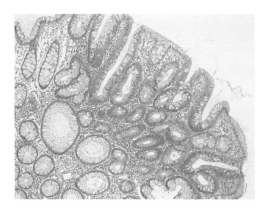

Figure 14.80 Adenomatous polyp with low-grade dysplasia (corresponds to Figures 14.75–14.79) (Hospital Sao Marcos).

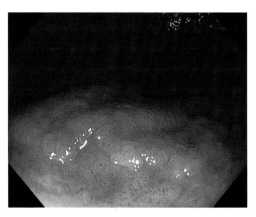

Figure 14.81 Flat adenoma in cecum with NBI showing 3L pits (Indiana University School of Medicine).

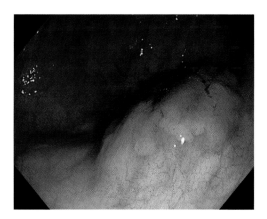

Figure 14.82 White light HRE view of flat adenoma in the cecum after submucosal injection with saline and methylene blue (corresponds to Figure 14.81) (Indiana University School of Medicine).

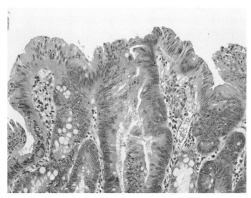

Figure 14.83 Portion of tubulovillous adenoma in high power (corresponds to Figures 14.81 and 14.82) (Indiana University School of Medicine).

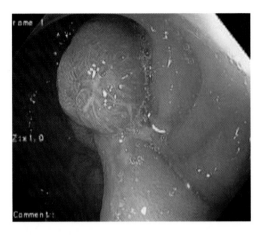

Figure 14.84 White light low-magnification view of pedunculated polyp (Catholic University of the Sacred Heart).

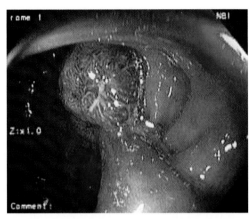

Figure 14.85 NBI view of pedunculated polyp (Catholic University of the Sacred Heart).

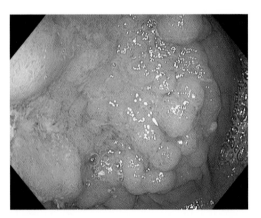

Figure 14.86 A 5 cm tubulovillous adenoma of the cecum (Mount Sinai School of Medicine).

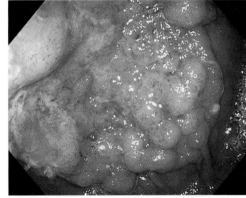

Figure 14.87 A 5 cm tubulovillous adenoma of the cecum (NBI image) (corresponds to Figures 14.86–14.90) (Mount Sinai School of Medicine).

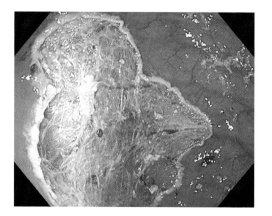

Figure 14.88 A 5 cm tubulovillous adenoma of the cecum after removal by piecemeal polypectomy (Mount Sinai School of Medicine).

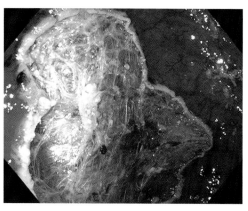

Figure 14.89 A 5 cm tubulovillous adenoma of the cecum after removal by piecemeal polypectomy (NBI image) (Mount Sinai School of Medicine).

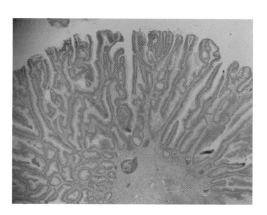

Figure 14.90 A 5 cm tubulovillous adenoma of the cecum (path) (corresponds to Figures 14.86–14.89) (Mount Sinai School of Medicine).

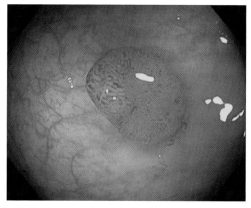

Figure 14.91 White light low-magnification view of colonic polyp (corresponds to Figure 14.92) (Institut Arnault Tzanck).

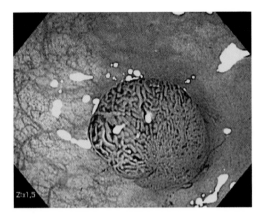

Figure 14.92 NBI view of colonic adenoma with 1.5× magnification. Pit pattern and vessel pattern consistent with pathological diagnosis of tubulovillous adenoma (corresponds to Figure 14.91) (Institut Arnault Tzanck).

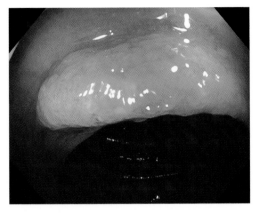

Figure 14.93 HRE white light low-magnification view of villous adenoma on a fold (University of Utah Health Sciences Center).

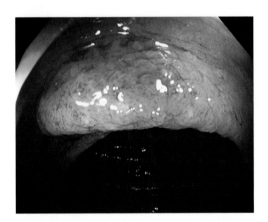

Figure 14.94 NBI light view of a villous adenoma. Note the typical villiform and sulcated surface appearance (corresponds to Figure 14.93) (University of Utah Health Sciences Center).

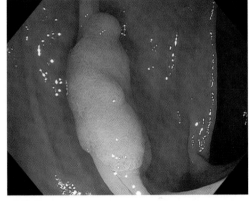

Figure 14.95 White light image of tubulovillous adenoma in transverse colon with focal high-grade dysplasia (corresponds to Figures 14.96 and 14.97) (Indiana University School of Medicine).

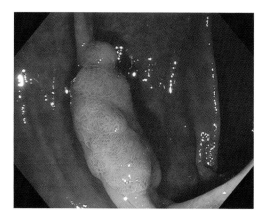

Figure 14.96 NBI image of tubulovillous adenoma in the transverse colon with focal high-grade dysplasia and type 3L and 4 pits (Indiana University School of Medicine).

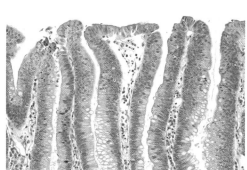

Figure 14.97 Tubulovillous adenoma in transverse colon with focal high-grade dysplasia in high power (corresponds to Figures 14.95 and 14.96) (Indiana University School of Medicine).

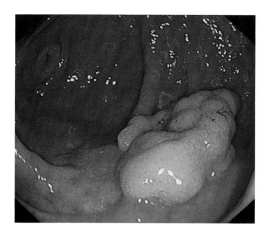

Figure 14.98 Large sessile colon polyp seen here in low-magnification white light. Histology after endoscopic resection revealed a tubulovillous adenoma with free resection margins (University of Amsterdam).

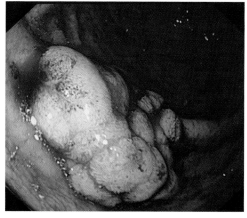

Figure 14.99 Chromoendoscopy with methylene blue nicely reveals the borders of the lesion in preparation for polypectomy (corresponds to Figures 14.98–14.100) (University of Amsterdam).

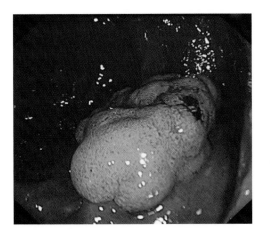

Figure 14.100 Low-magnification NBI view of the polyp also provides excellent demarcation of the border comparable to chromoendoscopy (corresponds to Figures 14.98–14.99) (University of Amsterdam).

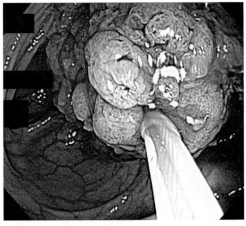

Figure 14.101 This non-HRE white light view of a giant tubulovillous colon adenoma undergoing piecemeal snare polypectomy after tattooing. Note the difference in resolution with the subsequent HRE images taken for the follow-up examination (corresponds to Figures 14.102–14.105) (NYU School of Medicine).

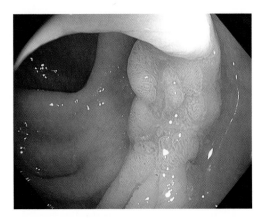

Figure 14.102 White light HRE easily identifies the site of scar and residual polyp 5 weeks following near complete piecemeal resection of 6cm tubulovillous adenoma with APC fulguration (NYU School of Medicine).

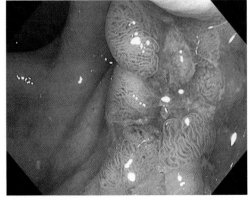

Figure 14.103 NBI low-magnification view shows central scar and villous adenoma pit pattern in this residual lesion. Pathology confirmed residual tubulovillous adenoma (NYU School of Medicine).

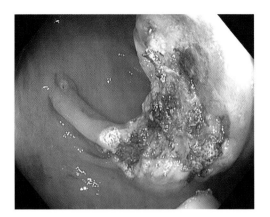

Figure 14.104 White light HRE view of lesion following snare resection and APC fulguration (NYU School of Medicine).

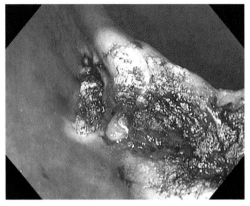

Figure 14.105 NBI low-magnification view of the lesion following snare resection and APC fulguration. No residual polypoid tissue is visualized (corresponds to Figures 14.101–14.104) (NYU School of Medicine).

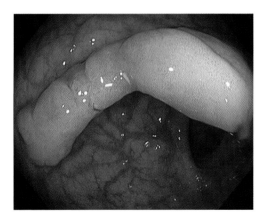

Figure 14.106 White light low-magnification image of tubular adenoma (Indiana University School of Medicine).

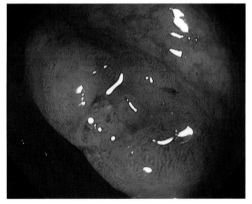

Figure 14.107 NBI image of tubular adenoma with high-grade dysplasia (corresponds to Figures 14.106 and 14.108) (Indiana University School of Medicine).

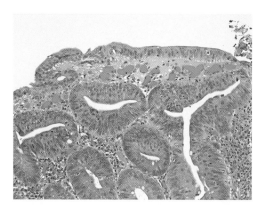

Figure 14.108 Tubular adenoma with high-grade dysplasia in high power (corresponds to Figures 14.106 and 14.107) (Indiana University School of Medicine).

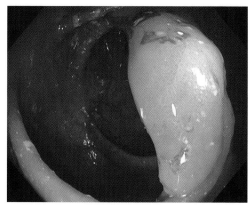

Figure 14.109 White light image of a tubulovillous adenoma with low-grade dysplasia in the transverse colon (Indiana University School of Medicine).

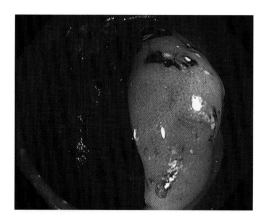

Figure 14.110 NBI image of tubulovillous adenoma in the transverse colon with low-grade dysplasia. Note type 3L and 4 pits (Indiana University School of Medicine).

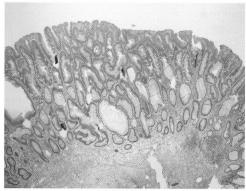

Figure 14.111 Tubulovillous adenoma in low power (corresponds to Figures 14.109 and 14.110) (Indiana University School of Medicine).

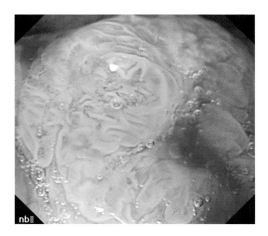

Figure 14.112 Magnified HRE view of colon adenocarcinoma. (Institut Arnault Tzanck).

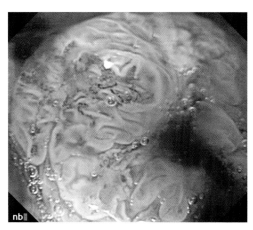

Figure 14.113 NBI magnification view of intramucosal adenocarcinoma. Note the area of frank malignancy showing completely distorted pit pattern (corresponds to Figure 14.112) (Institut Arnault Tzanck).

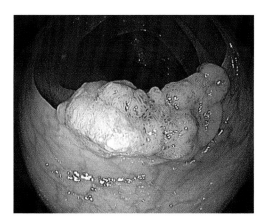

Figure 14.114 White light low-magnification view of a laterally spreading colon tumor (Institut Arnault Tzanck).

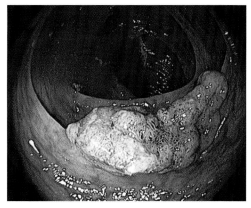

Figure 14.115 NBI low-magnification view of the same lesion (corresponds to Figure 14.114) (Institut Arnault Tzanck).

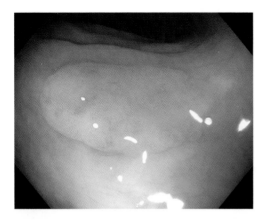

Figure 14.116 Typical appearance of a serrated adenoma with the appearance of an accentuated fold. The architecture is indistinct on this white light view (University of Utah Health Sciences Center).

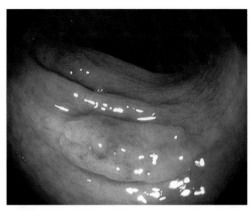

Figure 14.117 Typical appearance of a serrated adenoma with the appearance of an accentuated fold seen with NBI light. The architecture is somewhat pitted with villiform components and is better defined than on the white light view (University of Utah Health Sciences Center).

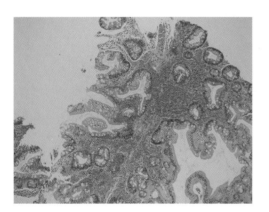

Figure 14.118 Colonic mucosa with hyperplastic glands having a "sawtooth" appearance at the surface and dilation at the base with basal goblet cells. No dysplasia is seen (corresponds to Figures 14.116 and 14.117) (University of Utah Health Sciences Center).

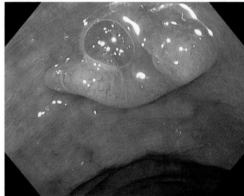

Figure 14.119 NBI non-magnified view of a sessile polyp with a mixed surface vascular pattern found on pathology to be a serrated polyp (NYU School of Medicine).

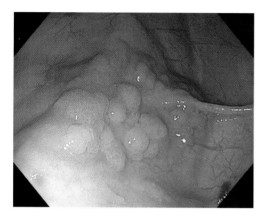

Figure 14.120 Laterally spreading adenoma in cecum (Mount Sinai School of Medicine).

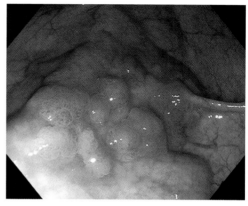

Figure 14.121 NBI low magnification view of lateral spreading adenoma in the cecum (corresponds to Figures 14.120–14.126) (Mount Sinai School of Medicine).

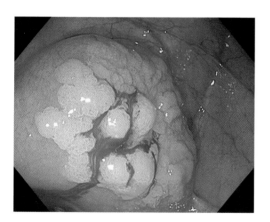

Figure 14.122 Cecal adenoma elevated on pillow of saline from submucosal injection prior to piecemeal resection (Mount Sinai School of Medicine).

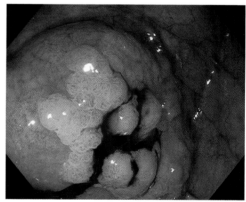

Figure 14.123 NBI view of the cecal adenoma following submucosal injection of saline (Mount Sinai School of Medicine).

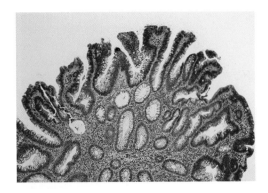

Figure 14.124 Laterally spreading adenoma in cecum (path) (corresponds to Figures 14.120–14.123) (Mount Sinai School of Medicine).

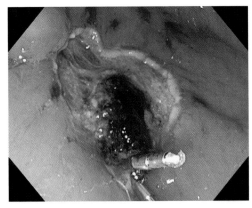

Figure 14.125 Post-polypectomy site after APC and clips. Polypectomy done under white light. NBI used afterwards to rule out residual polyp (corresponds to Figures 14.120–14.126) (Mount Sinai School of Medicine).

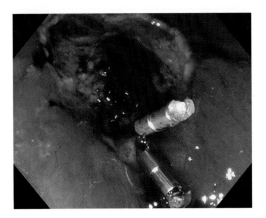

Figure 14.126 NBI view of polyp site following piecemeal resection and APC with two clips for hemostasis; no residual polyp present (Mount Sinai School of Medicine).

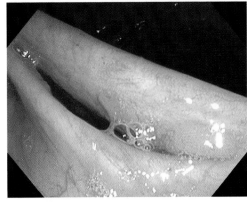

Figure 14.127 White light view with barely apparent polyps on the lip of the ileocecal valve (corresponds to Figures 14.128–14.130) (Mount Sinai School of Medicine).

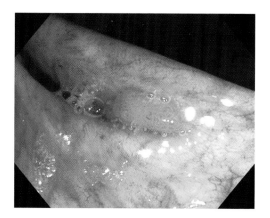

Figure 14.128 NBI low-magnification view of two polyps on the lip of the ileocecal valve (corresponds to Figures 14.127–14.130) (Mount Sinai School of Medicine).

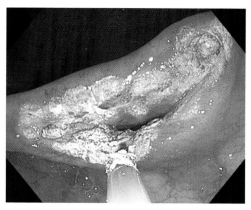

Figure 14.129 APC fulguration of polyps on lip of ileocecal valve (Mount Sinai School of Medicine).

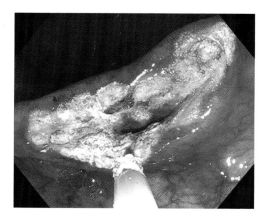

Figure 14.130 NBI view of APC fulguration of polyps on ileocecal valve (corresponds to Figures 14.127–14.129) (Mount Sinai School of Medicine).

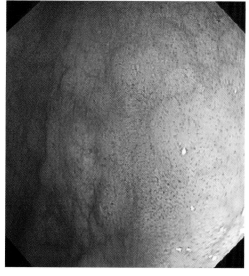

Figure 14.131 Multiple rectal adenomas in FAP (corresponds to Figure 14.132) (St. Mark's Hospital).

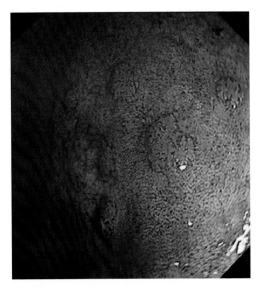

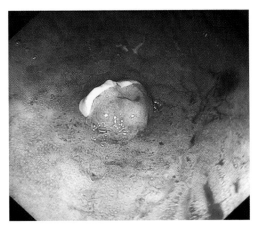

Figure 14.133 Inflammatory polyp in ulcerative colitis with fibrin cap (St. Mark's Hospital).

Figure 14.132 Multiple adenomas in FAP. Note with NBI improved contrast for adenoma edges (corresponds to Figure 14.131) (St. Mark's Hospital).

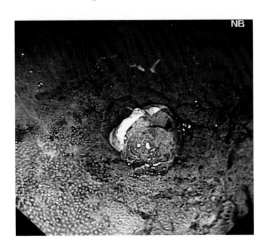

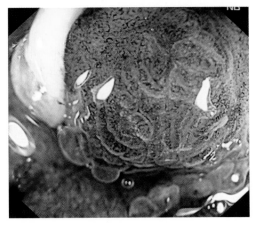

Figure 14.134 Inflammatory polyp in ulcerative colitis with NBI. Pit pattern and fibrin cap are well seen (corresponds to Figure 14.133) (St. Mark's Hospital).

Figure 14.135 Magnification NBI view of inflammatory polyp in ulcerative colitis with pseudo type 4 pit pattern. However, histopathology reveals mainly granulation tissue (corresponds to Figures 14.133 and 14.134) (St. Mark's Hospital).

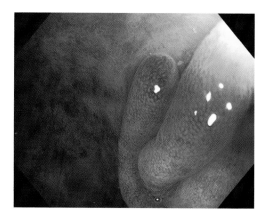

Figure 14.136 Classic psudopolyps in an area of mild inflammation in chronic ulcerative colitis, NBI non-magnification view (NYU School of Medicine).

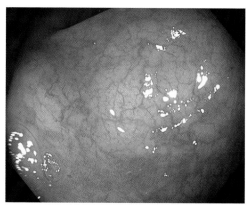

Figure 14.137 Mild erythema and small superficial erosions in active chronic colitis white light non-magnified view (NYU School of Medicine).

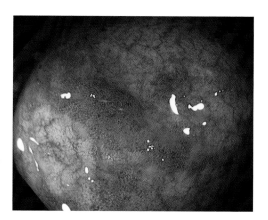

Figure 14.138 Active chronic colitis NBI low-magnification view (NYU School of Medicine).

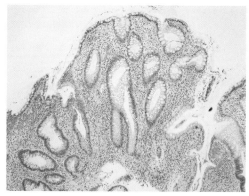

Figure 14.139 Active chronic ulcerative colitis. The mucosal architecture is distorted with branched glands and abnormal gland spacing, and a mixed acute and chronic inflammatory infiltrate expands the mucosa (corresponds to Figures 14.137–14.138) (NYU School of Medicine) .

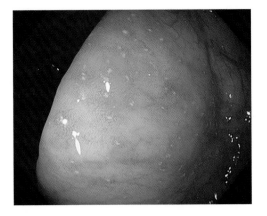

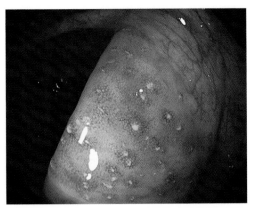

Figure 14.140 White light view of punctate erosions in the cecum of a patient with ulcerative colitis (NYU School of Medicine).

Figure 14.141 NBI low-magnification view of punctate cecal erosions in this patient with mildly active ulcerative colitis (NYU School of Medicine).

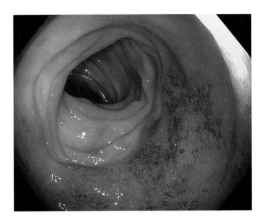

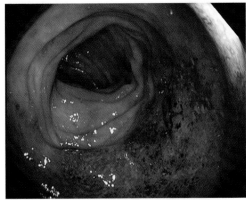

Figure 14.142 Sharp demarcation of inflammation from normal mucosa at the splenic flexure in this patient with left-sided ulcerative colitis (University of Utah Health Sciences Center).

Figure 14.143 An NBI light view of a sharp demarcation between inflammated and normal mucosa at the splenic flexure (University of Utah Health Sciences Center).

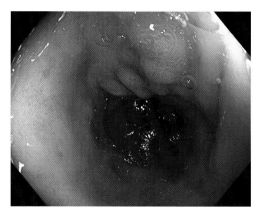

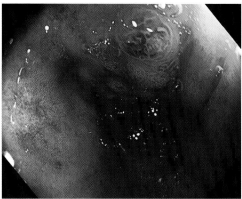

Figure 14.144 Polypoid area in sigmoid colon of patient with ulcerative colitis in remission (NYU School of Medicine).

Figure 14.145 High-magnification NBI image of polypoid lesion with irregular vascular pattern and villous appearing sulci in a patient with chronic ulcerative colitis in remission (NYU School of Medicine).

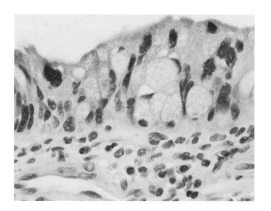

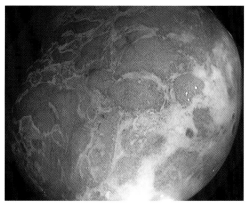

Figure 14.146 High-grade dysplasia in ulcerative colitis. There is loss of polarity in the surface epithelial cells, some of which contain atypical, enlarged hyperchromatic nuclei (corresponds to Figures 14.144 and 14.145) (NYU School of Medicine).

Figure 14.147 Active rectal superficial ulceration with focal polypoid area (corresponds to Figures 14.148 and 14.149) (NYU School of Medicine).

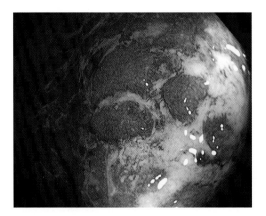

Figure 14.148 Low magnification NBI view of the focal polypoid area in this patient with active rectal ulceration. (corresponds to Figures 14.147 and 14.149) (NYU School of Medicine).

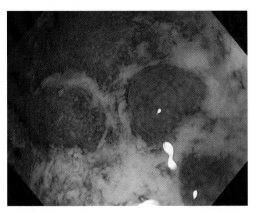

Figure 14.149 High magnification NBI view of the raised bump in this patient that, in contrast to the raised dysplastic lesion in Figures 14.144 and 14.145, shows a regular mucosal pit pattern and normal vessels. Pathology revealed only inflammatory changes (NYU School of Medicine).

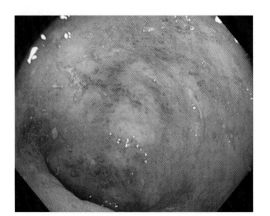

Figure 14.150 Active ulcerative colitis, white light low-magnification view (Institut Arnault Tzanck).

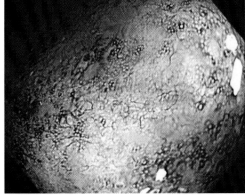

Figure 14.151 NBI view of the same area more clearly shows the vascular pattern associated with active inflammation (corresponds to Figure 14.150) (Institut Arnault Tzanck).

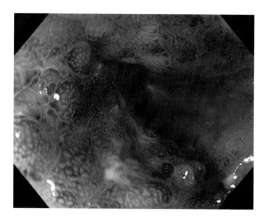

Figure 14.152 HGIN in ulcerative colitis 38-year-old female with 19-year history of ulcerative colitis. Depressed area with villous pattern (University Medical Center Hamburg Eppendorf).

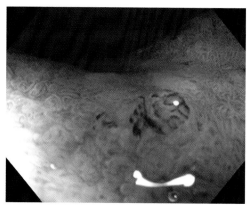

Figure 14.153 HGIN and LGIN in long-term ulcerative colitis, image taken from the nearest distance. Elevated area with gyrus-like pattern was HGIN, the surrounding villous area was LGIN (University Medical Center Hamburg Eppendorf).

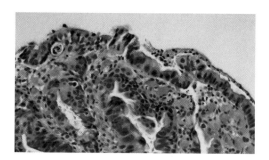

Figure 14.154 Gyriform area in the rectum, HGIN. Surrounding villous tissue (not shown) demonstrated LGIN from the same lesion. Neoplastic glands show highly enlarged rounded nuclei with prominent nucleoli (corresponds to Figure 14.153) (University Medical Center Hamburg Eppendorf).

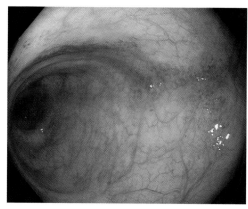

Figure 14.155 White light view of mild colitis due to Crohn's disease with a patchy erythematous appearance (corresponds to Figure 14.156) (University of Utah Health Sciences Center).

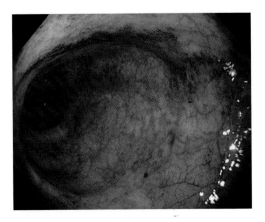

Figure 14.156 NBI light view of mild Crohn's colitis with the patch erythematous area seen as dark discoloration (corresponds to Figure 14.155) (University of Utah Health Sciences Center).

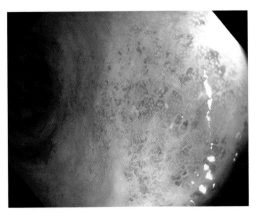

Figure 14.157 White light view of moderate Crohn's colitis with erythema and crypt distortion (University of Utah Health Sciences Center).

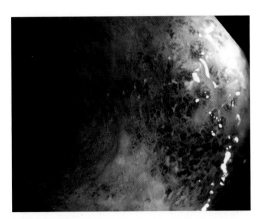

Figure 14.158 NBI light view of moderate Crohn's colitis with the inflamed areas seen in dark green (corresponds to Figure 14.157) (University of Utah Health Sciences Center).

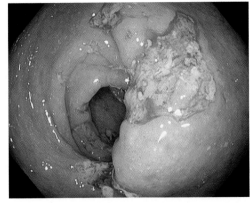

Figure 14.159 Ulcerated cecum in a patient with confirmed celiac disease and ASCA positive Crohn's disease (corresponds to Figures 14.160 and 14.161) (NYU School of Medicine).

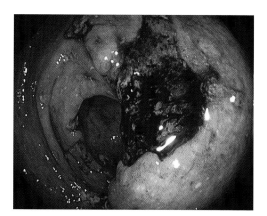

Figure 14.160 NBI view of ulcerated cecum in a patient with confirmed celiac disease and ASCA positive Crohn's disease (corresponds to Figures 14.159 and 14.161) (NYU School of Medicine).

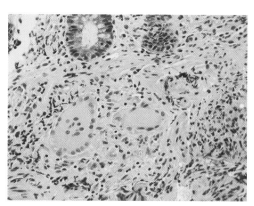

Figure 14.161 Granulomatous colitis in Crohn's disease. A non-necrotizing granuloma containing multinucleate giant cells is present at the base of the mucosa (corresponds to Figures 14.159 and 14.160) (NYU School of Medicine).

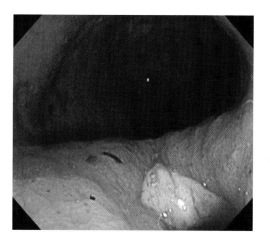

Figure 14.162 Colonic ulcer in Crohn's disease (Mount Sinai School of Medicine).

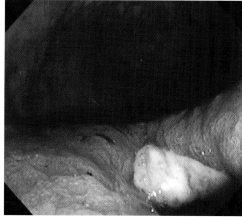

Figure 14.163 Colonic ulcer in Crohn's disease (NBI image) (Mount Sinai School of Medicine).

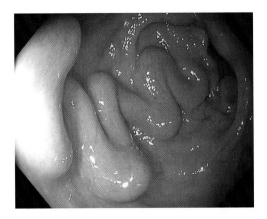

Figure 14.164 Tortuous rectal varix under white light low-magnification HRE view (NYU School of Medicine).

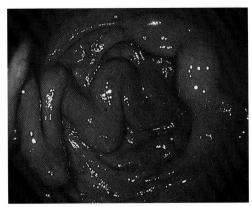

Figure 14.165 Low-magnification NBI view of tortuous rectal varix (NYU School of Medicine).

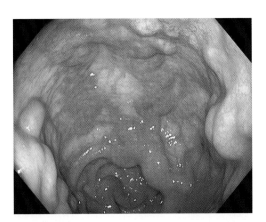

Figure 14.166 Multiple non-bleeding rectal varices seen on white light low-magnification HRE (NYU School of Medicine).

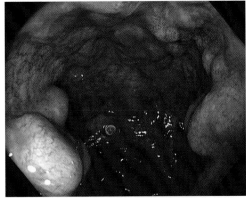

Figure 14.167 Multiple non-bleeding rectal varices seen in NBI low-magnified view (NYU School of Medicine).

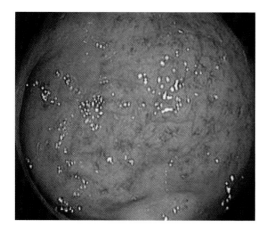

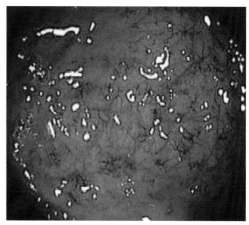

Figure 14.168 Endoscopic view of radiation proctitis (Catholic University of the Sacred Heart).

Figure 14.169 NBI view of radiation proctitis (Catholic University of the Sacred Heart).

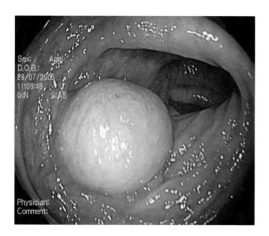

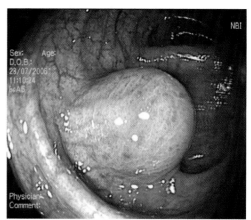

Figure 14.170 White light HRE view of colon lipoma (Hospital Sao Marcos).

Figure 14.171 NBI image of colon lipoma (Hospital Sao Marcos).

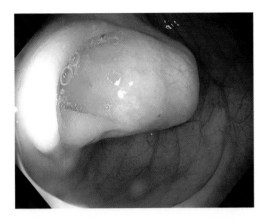

Figure 14.172 This large smooth apparent submucosal nodule seen next to the appendiceal orifice here in white light HRE (NYU School of Medicine).

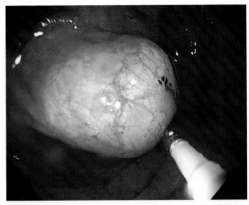

Figure 14.173 NBI view of this lesion which was felt to be firm and without pillowing upon probing with closed biopsy forceps (NYU School of Medicine).

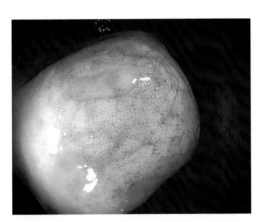

Figure 14.174 Magnification 1.5× NBI view of this suspected submucosal nodule confirms normal colon mucosal pit pattern (corresponds to Figures 14.172–14.173) (NYU School of Medicine).

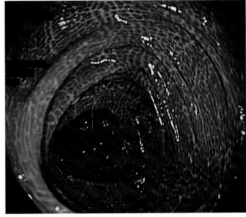

Figure 14.175 NBI non-magnified view of melanosis coli (corresponds to Figure 14.176) (Hospital Sao Marcos).

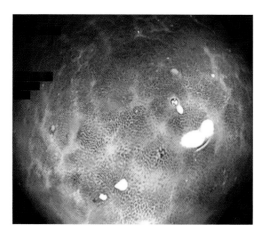

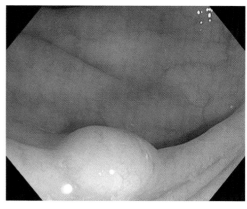

Figure 14.176 Melanosis coli, magnified NBI view (corresponds to Figure 14.175) (Hospital Sao Marcos).

Figure 14.177 A 3 mm submucosal mass in sigmoid – pathology shows low-grade carcinoid (Mount Sinai School of Medicine).

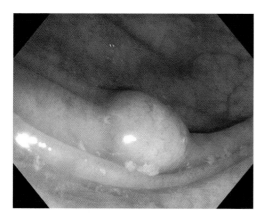

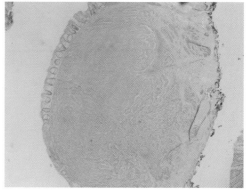

Figure 14.178 A 3 mm submucosal carcinoid in sigmoid – NBI confirms normal overyling mucosa (Mount Sinai School of Medicine).

Figure 14.179 A 3 mm submucosal mass in sigmoid – pathology shows low-grade carcinoid (corresponds to Figures 14.177–14.178) (Mount Sinai School of Medicine).

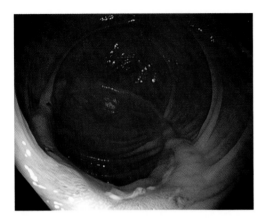

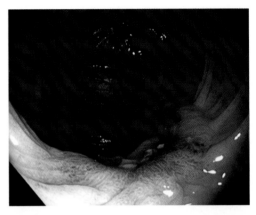

Figure 14.180 Ischemic ulcer of the cecum, white light HRE view. Note the linear ulcer with a white base (University of Utah Health Sciences Center).

Figure 14.181 Ischemic ulcer of the cecum viewed with NBI light (University of Utah Health Sciences Center).

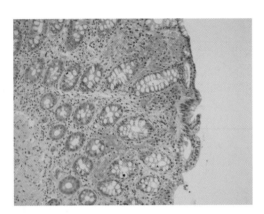

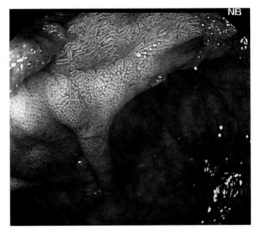

Figure 14.182 The photos depict colonic mucosa with eosinophilia of the lamina propria, mild crypt atrophy, and focal mucosal hemorrhage, with 20× magnification (corresponds to Figures 14.180 and 14.181) (University of Utah Health Sciences Center).

Figure 14.183 Ileocolonic anastomosis low-magnification NBI view (St. Mark's Hospital).

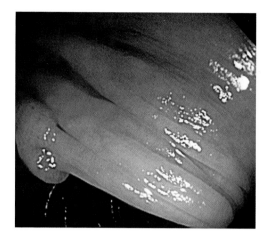

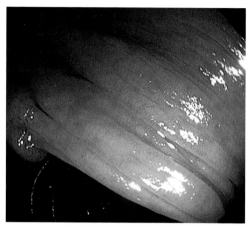

Figure 14.184 Prior India ink tatoo with polyp partially hidden behind a fold (Mount Sinai School of Medicine).

Figure 14.185 Prior India ink tatoo mark less visible on NBI non-magnified view. Polyp partially behind fold (Mount Sinai School of Medicine).

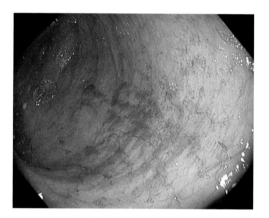

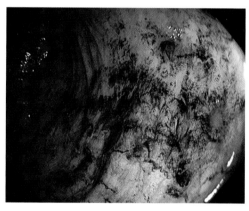

Figure 14.186 Numerous angioectasias of proximal colon with mild oozing, white light view (NYU School of Medicine).

Figure 14.187 NBI low-magnification view of proximal colon angioectasias (NYU School of Medicine).

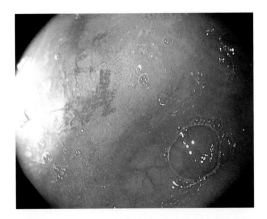

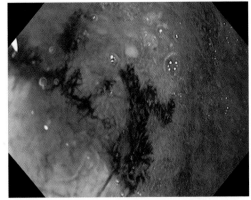

Figure 14.188 Non-magnified white light HRE view of a cecal angioectasia (NYU School of Medicine).

Figure 14.189 Magnified 1.5× NBI image of cecal angioectasia (NYU School of Medicine).

ABBREVIATIONS USED

APC: adenomatous polyposis coli
ASCA: anti-*Saccharomyces cerevisiae* antibodies
FAP: familial adenomatous polyposis
HGIN: high-grade intraepithelial neoplasia
LGIN: low-grade intraepithelial neoplasia
HRE: high-resolution endoscopy
NBI: narrowband imaging

Index

Note: page numbers in *italics* represent figures, those in **bold** represent tables.